S0-CEZ-152

Praise for Annie Hopper and
*Wired for Healing: Remapping the Brain to Recover
from Chronic and Mysterious Illnesses*

WHAT DOCTORS SAY:

*"Annie Hopper weaves together cutting-edge scientific research
based on neurological rehabilitation and functional imaging, with
the age-old traditions of mindfulness and healing. Her program
has the potential to significantly dampen inflammatory conditions
and, perhaps more importantly, encourage self-empowerment."*

— Dr. Cynthia Li, MD,
    Internal Medicine,
    Berkeley, CA

*"Annie Hopper's program, which addresses the limbic system
"engrained memory" aspect of Multiple Chemical Sensitivity
and many other conditions, is the only way I've found for some
patients to get out of their illnesses. Physical treatment is often
just not enough. ...there are now patients I won't even begin to
treat until they go through her program."*

— Dr. William Shrader, MD,
    Environmental Medicine,
    Santa Fe, NM

*"Annie Hopper understands that in order for our brains to cope
with the world, the 'feeling', 'thinking', 'integrating' and 'doing'
circuits need to talk to each other. Annie Hopper understands these
principles, and, as her work demonstrates, is able to use these in a
practical and sensible manner, in a way that resonates. Her work
enables our brains to become more efficient communicators, not
only with ourselves but with the world around us. Read this book!"*

— Dr. Les Koopowitz, MBBCh, FFPsych (SA),
    Clinical Associate Professor in Psychiatry
    University of Adelaide, Practising in Neuropsychiatry

WHAT PATIENTS SAY:

"I am shaking my head and pinching myself and overcome with gratitude. Wow!!! I am getting my life back!"
> — Jessica suffered from chronic fatigue syndrome, multiple chemical sensitivities, food sensitivities and other chronic conditions that rendered her disabled for 6 years.

"In 2011, I went from being an active and happy Mom to being bedridden. I was completely homebound, unable to function and was pretty much miserable ALL the time. I'M SO HAPPY that I have made such lasting improvements with the program. THANK YOU SO MUCH!!"
> — Jared had suffered from postural orthostatic tachycardia syndrome, chemical, electrical, and food sensitivities, mast cell activation disorder, and Hashimotos syndrome for 4 years.

"The limbic system is sensitive to trauma and we have suffered from injury to the limbic system in the brain – and this program is the appropriate treatment. It's the best treatment — it works!"
> — Judy suffered from chronic fatigue syndrome and multiple chemical sensitivities for 21 years.

"I experienced moderate MCS, EHS, and Food Sensitivities for five years and within seven months this has turned around. This has decreased the stress on my entire family and I feel that I have a life again!"
> — Layna suffered from food sensitivities, electric hypersensitivity syndrome and multiple chemical sensitivities for 5 years.

"I would ask people to have courage and make the change. This will be the start of a complete new life. You can do it. I have."
> — Narguis sufferered from chronic pain, anxiety and multiple chemical sensitivities for 20 years.

"This is the catalyst for change that you are looking for....I am 98% better from Food Sensitivities. I eat everything except for two (kinds of) nuts."
> — Erin suffered from food sensitivities and multiple chemical sensitivities for 20 years.

"I cannot believe the changes in my life. I go anywhere and do anything. I just want to say that this program saved my life, my relationship with family, partner, friends etc. Thank you Annie for what you have done for me and for the countless sufferers out there in no persons land. When I first got sick, I wanted to kill myself – but there was a voice inside that said don't – thank God I listened to the voice. Life is good today!" "This program really saved my life... there is nothing that I am not doing in my life today. Nothing... It is a miracle."

— Andrea suffered from electric hypersensitivity syndrome and multiple chemical sensitivities for 2 years.

"Even though I'm a Registered Nurse and we learned about the limbic system; I never thought that this was causing all of the problems."

— Judy suffered from severe food sensitivities, chronic fatigue syndrome, fibromyalgia and multiple chemical sensitivities for 17 years.

"I am so happy and excited about my future! Annie needs to be cloned so she can be in more places! I just thought you should know how grateful I am!"

— Kathleen suffered from chronic fatigue syndrome and multiple chemical sensitivities for 6 years.

WIRED FOR HEALING:

Remapping the Brain to Recover from Chronic and Mysterious Illnesses

Annie Hopper

Wired for Healing: Remapping the Brain to Recover from
Chronic and Mysterious Illnesses
©2014 The Dynamic Neural Retraining System™

All rights reserved worldwide. No part of this publication may be copied, modified, reproduced, transmitted, or translated in any form or by any means, electronic, mechanic, recording, or otherwise, without express written permission from Annie Hopper. This publication cannot be used to tailor products, create new products or derivative works in any written, visual, or audio form, or by any means electronic or mechanical.

Cover design by James Tozer

Cover artwork by Christine Crossley www.artfulwaves.com

Author photo by Ian Redd Photography

Typeset in *Aldus* with *Baker* display at SpicaBookDesign

Paperback ISBN 978-0-9938901-0-9

Published by The Dynamic Neural Retraining System™
Victoria, B.C. Canada

As a company, the Dynamic Neural Retraining System™ is very passionate about the environment and we take an active role in promoting environmental awareness. We believe in the importance of caring for people, caring for the planet, and caring for all of its inhabitants. We think this makes good business sense and is simply the right thing to do. With these values in mind, we are committed in our mission to create healthy products that have minimal environmental impact. This book is printed on acid-free paper that is 100% old growth forest-free (100% post-consumer recycled), processed chlorine free, and printed with vegetable, low-VOC inks.

For further information or to browse our complete list of products and purchase securely, visit our website at www.retrainingthebrain.com

Printed in Canada by Friesens
2nd printing May 2016
3rd printing April 2017

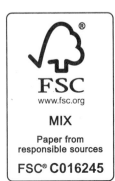

FSC
www.fsc.org
MIX
Paper from
responsible sources
FSC® C016245

ENVIRONMENTAL BENEFITS STATEMENT

Annie Hopper saved the following resources by printing the pages of this book on chlorine free paper made with 100% post-consumer waste.

TREES	WATER	ENERGY	SOLID WASTE	GREENHOUSE GASES
21	9,592	9	642	1,768
FULLY GROWN	GALLONS	MILLION BTUs	POUNDS	POUNDS

Environmental impact estimates were made using the Environmental Paper Network Paper Calculator 3.2. For more information visit www.papercalculator.org.

This book is dedicated to my mother
Agnes Genevieve Hopper

…..thank you for always believing in me.

Note to the Reader

While the stories of the individuals featured in this book are true, I have modified or used their first name only in order to protect their privacy.

The Dynamic Neural Retraining System™ (DNRS)

The Dynamic Neural Retraining System™ helps restore normal limbic system function in patients suffering from multiple chemical sensitivities, chronic fatigue syndrome, fibromyalgia, electric hypersensitivity syndrome, mould sensitivity, food, light and sound sensitivities, depression, anxiety, Gulf War Syndrome, post traumatic stress disorder, postural orthostatic tachycardia syndrome, chronic pain, irritable bowel syndrome and a host of other chronic and inflammatory conditions. It is a top-down neuroplasticity-based psychoneuroimmunological intervention that assists in normalizing the threat and survival mechanism within the limbic system and downgrades the brain's maladapted chronic stress response.

According to the Statistics Canada 2010 Canadian Community Health Survey, it was estimated that 1.4 million people suffered from chronic fatigue syndrome (CFS), fibromyalgia or multiple chemical sensitivities (MCS) in Canada alone. The current total population of Canada is approximately 35 million, whereas the United States population is approximately 317 million. If the rates of occurrence for these conditions in Canada are comparable to the U.S., then it would be reasonable to estimate at least 13 million people in the U.S. currently suffer from these conditions. Some of the latest research suggests that 22% of individuals with chronic health issues suffer from some degree of chemical intolerance (Katerndahl, D. A., Bell, I. R., Palmer, R. F., and Miller, C. S. 2012).

The Dynamic Neural Retraining System™ is a drug free, self-directed, neuroplasticity-based treatment that is taught from a platform of environmental awareness. This intensive program is experiential in nature and focuses on normalizing the threat and survival mechanism within the limbic system of the brain. The program integrates components of cognitive behaviour therapy, mindfulness based cognitive restructuring, emotional restructuring therapy, neural linguistic programming, incremental exposure and behaviour modification therapy.

This mechanism-targeted behavioural intervention is based in an affect-science perspective, and focuses on the training of a number of regulatory skills including attention focusing, attention distraction, cognitive reappraisal, emotional distancing, emotion regulation as well as experiential and incremental exposure therapy to contexts of perceived risk.

The DNRS program examines how various forms of trauma can affect the stress and protective mechanisms in the brain, how trauma can manifest itself on physical, psychological, and emotional levels, and how these affect overall health. Patients learn how to effectively interrupt the maladapted 'fight-or-flight' stress response and stop the flood of stress-initiated biochemicals that activate cytokine activity and inflammation. Patients also learn to remap the neural circuits that influence survival and stress mechanisms, thereby normalizing sensory perception, detoxification, immune function, and inflammatory responses. This works to prevent numerous downstream effects through the hypothalamus-pituitary-adrenal axis, such as hormonal dysregulation and immune system dysfunction. Once the limbic system is calm, parasympathetic nervous system balance resumes, allowing for more restful sleep, cellular detoxification, and restoration of intestinal permeability. Pain signal processing and other forms of distorted sensory perception are also normalized. This effectively increases energy and well-being and decreases many symptoms of illness involving distorted sensory perception.

COMPANY VISION

The Dynamic Neural Retraining System™ endeavours to:

- Provide tools for healing to people suffering from limbic system impairments.
- Promote awareness of limbic system-related conditions.
- Provide medical practitioners and medical educational systems with the information and tools to effectively diagnose, refer and treat patients.
- Promote awareness of the negative effects of environmental toxins on brain function.
- Promote environmental awareness as a means to prevent illness.
- Provide access to programs by creating treatment centres globally, beginning in Canada and the United States.

As a company, we are very passionate about the environment and take an active role in promoting environmental awareness. We believe in the importance of caring for people, caring for the planet, and caring for all of its inhabitants. With these values in mind, we are committed in our mission to create healthy products that have minimal environmental impact. We think this makes good business sense and is simply the right thing to do.

Having successfully treated limbic system conditions since 2008, we are familiar with the effects of toxic trauma on the brain and the rehabilitation process, and we look forward to continuing our global outreach in the years to come.

Acknowledgements

When I was sick and living on a broken down houseboat, I made a promise to myself that, when and if I found a way out of illness, I would share this information in the best possible way with the world. I believe that I have done the best that I can in this respect, but it would not have been possible without the help and support of many people. I want to take this opportunity to personally thank my amazing team of people who have graciously helped me with this task.

Perhaps the most influential person in my life to date is my partner James Tozer. When you read the story of our relationship, you will understand why. In order to accurately convey what I have learned being in relationship with James would require another book. Perhaps I will write it some day, but for now what I will share with you is that we have learned a great deal about love, life and neuroplasticity together.

To James, your love and support is the stepping-stone for my ability to reach others and an invaluable contribution to our work in this world. Without you, I simply could not do what I do. Your support is not only measured in our quality of life, but in the lives that we touch through our work. I know that you are sincerely the happiest when you are serving humanity and I'm so glad that we get to work together and share our gifts with the world in this unique way. I am so blessed to share this journey with you.

To my Mum, thanks for your continuous belief in me and for your unwavering love and support. You never questioned the severity of my illness; you were willing to make the concessions necessary to be with me, you prayed for me daily and you always loved me unconditionally. To my associate, Candy Widdifield, thank you for your invaluable contribution to the DNRS Team, for your insight and for being a soul sister on this journey. To Anna Malkin, thank you for helping me find the words that could adequately convey the message and for putting my thoughts into a format that makes sense. To Rick J. Goulden thank you for your editing assistance. To my brother Tom and my sister Barb, thank you also for your love, friendship and support. To the rest of the DNRS team, my assistant Jacqui Boone and DNRS Coaches Alita Hetland, Pat Parisi, and Lauren Dinkel – thank you for helping to support our clients in the best possible way. To my dog Bella, thank you for all of your cuddles and love and for your eternal playfulness. You are all such a blessing and gift to me. You are my greatest treasures and an invaluable part of this journey.

I would also like to thank all of the people who so graciously shared their stories of recovery with me. You are all true alchemists of your lives and a source of inspiration and hope for millions. Thank you for having the courage and discipline that is required to retrain your brain, transform your health and reclaim your life! May you always look at the world in the way you did when you were first able to do something as your renewed self. May your reverence for living your life to the fullest be with you for the rest of your days. May the feeling of gratitude for personal transformation always be close to your heart and remember that the problems you may face today are nothing when compared to what you have already lived through. Continue to share your story of transformation with as many people as possible; you never know who is almost ready to give up. Pray for those who still need healing. Continue to be a beacon of light and hope for the future, for humanity, and for the planet. The wisdom that you have gained through your journey is invaluable and is so needed in the world. I am blessed that our paths have crossed. Your stories of recovery fill my heart with love, and yes, tears of joy! Know that your story will give millions of people the hope and faith they need to believe that there is a better tomorrow.

Preface

I know what it's like to feel misunderstood and misdiagnosed by the medical system. For those of you who are suffering right now, I want you to know that you are not alone, that you are not crazy, and that it's not your fault. Limbic system-related illnesses such as multiple chemical sensitivities (MCS), also known as chemical intolerance (CI) and environmental illness (EI), fibromyalgia (FM), chronic fatigue syndrome (CFS), also known as myalgic encephalomyelitis (ME), electric hypersensitivity syndrome (EHS), chronic pain, food sensitivities, postural orthostatic tachycardia syndrome (POTS), post-traumatic stress disorder (PTSD), depression, irritable bowel syndrome, inflammatory conditions, Gulf War syndrome, and anxiety are not yet well understood. Information about brain function as it relates to these conditions is not common knowledge within the medical professions and may not be for some years to come. It is still relatively uncommon for your family doctor, a specialist, an allergist, an environmental doctor, a naturopath, or other alternative medical practitioner to properly diagnose or treat the underlying cause of your condition.

If you are suffering, you have likely gone from one treatment or practitioner to the next seeking relief from your symptoms, only to feel disappointed, disillusioned, and frustrated. When treatment attempts fail, you are left with dashed hopes, a deeper sense of hopelessness, helplessness, and growing skepticism about the possibility of recovery.

With the lack of validation from the medical industry, it is also quite common for your family, friends, and co-workers to perceive your illness as something that exists solely in your mind – something you made up or something you can control. Nothing could be further from the truth. Many of you are likely feeling like outcasts – isolated and abandoned by the people you thought would care for you the most. Please know that your suffering does not represent some kind of spiritual debt. Equally, you did not attract illness to you in any way, shape or form. Illness is also not the result of unresolved childhood wounds, nor is it the result of negative thoughts.

Limbic system dysfunction is located in the brain but the related conditions are far from being 'psychological' issues. They are trauma-induced brain impairments that affect many systems of the body. These conditions are physical in nature, they are real, they are painful, they are life altering, and they can be life threatening. Let me repeat: You are not alone, you are not crazy, and it's not your fault.

Simply put, all forms of trauma (physical, psychological, or emotional) have a profound affect on the brain, and can cause limbic system sensitization and dysfunction. Any trauma has the ability to activate deep limbic system circuits responsible for threat and protective mechanisms that affect both the brain and body.

How do I know that limbic system dysfunction is at the very heart of these conditions? Because I have suffered just as many of you are suffering now. I was completely disabled by severe multiple chemical sensitivities, fibromyalgia, and electric hypersensitivity syndrome. In fact, my symptoms were so severe that I became homeless, not for lack of money, but because my body was reacting to everyday chemicals and electromagnetic fields as if they were life threatening. The only place to find refuge was in nature, away from people, from chemicals, and from everything that made the symptoms worse. The pain was real, the suffering was real, and the isolation and sense of abandonment were also undeniably real.

If I had not experienced the suffering firsthand, I could not understand the illness or its progression today, nor would I be able to demonstrate to people how to heal themselves of these disabling limbic system-related conditions. Just like many of you, I had been to see countless doctors and specialists who could not help me. I spent my life savings on treatments that ultimately did not help. Some treatments seemed to be beneficial in the short term, but none were long lasting. In fact, some of the treatments that I tried were actually quite harmful and made my symptoms worse. Now that I understand limbic system dysfunction, I can see why my brain and body were not responding to treatments that may be beneficial for other people. Time and time again, I was left feeling hopeless and wondered if I would ever get out of the living nightmare, or if I would live at all! To be honest, my will to live at times was not very strong. This was surprising to me as I considered myself to be a very emotionally strong and stable person. Thoughts of ending my life were like dragons that I had to keep at bay, sometimes on a daily or hourly basis – just so that I did not have to endure another day of sickness, pain, and isolation. I can only imagine that the suicide rate among sufferers of this group of illnesses is very high and is largely unrecorded, as the majority of sufferers are misdiagnosed by the medical industry. Many don't know that their illness is a diagnosable condition. A limbic system disorder can bring even the healthiest people to their knees.

It was not until I addressed the illness as a physical brain injury that I could understand the illness and how to influence brain function. In hindsight, I am grateful that I was sick, as the journey has brought me to the very gracious position of helping others. In fact, other people often comment how glad they are that I personally experienced illness. Not that they wish me ill, but that they are grateful that someone has found a way out of the nightmare of a limbic system impairment after having experienced it personally.

When I was suffering, I made a promise to myself that if and when I recovered, I would do everything I could to assist others. In the beginning, this meant teaching my program in one of the only spaces I knew to be environmentally friendly enough for those who suffered from chemical sensitivities – the living room of my own home.

After recovering fully from the horrific experience of a limbic system injury, developing a recovery method that would help others recover just seemed like the right thing to do. As I continued on my quest to help those who were suffering, it became very evident to me that I would need to expand my ability to help people. Holding occasional programs could not meet the growing demand. I knew that there were many people that were afflicted with limbic system disorders who were suffering with such severe symptoms that it would literally make it impossible for them to attend a program in person. Daily I would receive numerous emails from people begging for help, and it broke my heart to continuously hear of such extreme suffering. I had to go back to the drawing board and find another way to disseminate the information.

In 2008, the Dynamic Neural Retraining System™ (DNRS) was launched to assist people in recovery from limbic system impairments. I knew that there were literally millions of people who were still suffering from debilitating conditions. Recent research shows that one in five people suffer from some kind of chemical intolerance, yet most physicians rarely diagnose this.

A July, 2012 article in the *Annals of Family Medicine* confirms these findings. In the report "Chemical Intolerance in Primary Care Settings: Prevalence, Comorbidity, and Outcomes," the authors reported that 20.3% of the patients studied met the criteria for chemical intolerance. (Katerndahl, D. A., Bell, I. R., Palmer, R. F., and Miller, C. S., 2012)

The physical involvement of the brain in these conditions is a relatively new understanding, yet it is integral to recovery. I believe that it is incredibly important for the medical industry to embrace this new information in order to refer patients to appropriate services even if it is outside of conventional practices.

With the understanding that not everyone would be able to attend an in-person program, we began to develop the instructional DVD set. In theory, this sounded like a good idea, although I had no idea how much work, time, or money that it would take to produce! Fortunately I am blessed with a fabulous support team who brought it all together. It was a huge amount of work, and the end product is a 14-hour instructional DVD. This set is now available in seven different languages, including a version with English subtitles for the hearing impaired. The DVD version was primarily created for people who cannot attend an in-person program due to illness restrictions.

We are often asked if the DVD is as effective as the in person program. Does it work? For some people, the DVD program will be enough to fully retrain their brain, and for others it will be a stepping stone to attending an in-person program. The DVD series gives people the science behind the program, the understanding necessary for the program to work, and the tools for recovery. The added benefit of the DVD set is that it can be viewed many times to enhance understanding of the program. Many people have fully recovered using the DVD set. The pivotal missing component of the DVD set is the experiential aspect of working with a group and with a certified DNRS instructor. For those who choose this method we highly recommend booking individual coaching to insure proper understanding and implementation of the program. Without working with each person, I cannot know if everyone has the correct understanding of the program, nor can I assess if everyone is implementing the information or the tools in the correct way.

The in-person program allows the patient to interact with their illness in a controlled environment. The group dynamic and the ongoing group support is an invaluable asset in the recovery process. The program includes neuroplasticity-based tools for redirecting brain function in a supportive group setting with one-on-one instruction. Participants have access to individual feedback and can tailor the program to suit their individual challenges and needs. A DNRS instructor helps the patient to discover any hidden obstacles to healing and assists the patient to work through challenges immediately. For many who have done both the DVD version and the live program, they say that the two cannot really be compared. The live program is by far the preferred option, but both methods complement each other.

The Dynamic Neural Retraining System™ has compiled data that demonstrate marked improvement and instances of full recovery from multiple chemical sensitivities over a six-month treatment period. A standardized research questionnaire was used to measure symptoms both before and after the Dynamic Neural Retraining System™ therapy.

In this book, I describe the function of the limbic system, the causes of dysfunction within the limbic system, and the ensuing physical, emotional, and psychological symptoms of dysfunction. I also discuss the basic concepts of the DNRS program and how it works to rewire the limbic system. I have also included a number of case studies. These incredibly hopeful and 'miraculous' stories of recovery are about real people and about the way they transformed their health using the DNRS program.

It is also imperative for the prevention of limbic system injury that we manage overall stress and become aware of the large array of environmental stressors that we are exposed to on a daily basis. With this in mind, I created the program with environmental awareness as a priority. Ultimately, this awareness will help us to decrease the overall toxic load on our brains and bodies and will prevent further injury and suffering.

For those of you who have patients with mysterious, multi-symptom illnesses that aren't responding to conventional or alternative treatment methods, please allow this book to introduce you to a new way of viewing this group of conditions. The brain's ability to change itself (neuroplasticity) greatly influences overall health and contributes to both the cause and resolution of many challenging illnesses. I invite you to view these case studies as an example of the power of neuroplasticity and to truly view the brain as the master organ of the body and source of optimal health.

Above all, my hope is that this book will serve as an avenue for understanding limbic system-related conditions, for renewed hope, and as a path of healing for those still suffering. You are not alone, your suffering has not been in vain, and you can live the life that you once dreamed of, even if you stopped dreaming a long time ago.

Introduction

In order to tell you where I am now, it is equally important to tell you where I came from and the influences that have brought me to this gracious place in life.

My partner James has also had a first-hand experience with neuroplasticity. He was profoundly deaf when we first met. He had lost some of his hearing at the age of five from a reaction to penicillin. His hearing started to deteriorate in a big way in his late twenties. By the time James was in his late thirties, he was classified as profoundly deaf. He was forty when we met, and, at that time, he could no longer use a phone or follow any live conversation due to his hearing impairment. Approximately two years after we started dating, James became the lucky recipient of a cochlear implant which gave him the ability to hear again. What this means is that sound was now being received through electrical impulses. In a nutshell, his brain had to relearn how to hear.

Two years after this, I had my own experience with neuroplasticity. I had suffered from a chemical brain injury that affected my limbic system, and my life quickly took a turn for the worse. Eventually, I did recover, which I will tell you all about in the next chapter.

Through it all, James was there. He stood by my side through my darkest hours, and, for this, I am eternally grateful. Now he works tirelessly at helping me deliver information to the world.

As I said, when we first met, James was profoundly deaf. Neither one of us knew sign language, and, because we were in a long distance relationship, we communicated mostly through emails to each other. When we were physically together I would communicate with James through writing via the computer or handwritten notes. I highly recommend this practice in general to get to know your loved ones. For me, it was important that James really knew me, and by that, I mean the inner me. As a core belief counsellor and as a person who deeply values personal awareness, I was accustomed to having conversations that revolved around these topics. Amongst my inner circle of friends, our conversations covered such topics as personal awareness, descriptions of our inner terrain, and an understanding of ourselves and the world around us. For me, this is still like poetry for my soul. For James, however, this was like speaking a foreign language. In order to share my world with him, I had to be creative and learn how to break down complex information about my internal world into smaller, bite-size pieces. I needed to convey my message in a written format that reflected common sense and describe my message with concrete and practical examples.

This skill set became invaluable later on when I started to write a newspaper column called "Emotional Rescue" for the *Kelowna Capital News*. In my column, I would write about general life challenges and describe their commonly associated inner terrain. I would elaborate on how to become an internal observer of one's inner self – how to identify emotions, thought processes, and resulting behaviour patterns. I would suggest ways to look at challenges from a different perspective, ways to foster compassion for self, and ways, through understanding and practical steps, to break habitual patterns in order to create a different outcome and avenues for greater understanding. Soon afterwards my column was also picked up by an Internet newspaper called Castanet.net.

Readers of my column would often comment on how my articles spoke directly to them. They would go so far as to clip the articles from the paper, collect them, or copy them and send them to their loved ones. My counselling practice grew tremendously as a result of this, and I was also invited to be a featured guest on local talk radio as an expert in emotional wellness.

Needless to say, my skill set of identifying and describing my inner terrain was invaluable during the recovery process from a limbic system injury. This has graciously allowed me to deliver a pivotal message of understanding limbic system dysfunction, the impact of the environment on brain function, and most importantly, the practical tools for recovery.

At one point during my journey with illness, I never could have imagined that I would be healthy again or successful again, nor could I have imagined that I would be in a position to help facilitate global healing or convey the importance of environmental awareness in this way. It never dawned on me that some day I would speak at brain injury conferences or speak to groups of medical doctors, educating them about limbic system dysfunction and the environment. In fact, there are times when I still do not feel like a proficient writer or a very eloquent speaker. I just know that I am an example of what it is like to suffer from a limbic system injury and that my experience and knowledge of rehabilitation can help millions of other people recover. This, I believe, is what I was born to do.

As it turns out, having the ability to relate my internal experience in an easily understood language, allowed me to communicate a greater message. I am extremely grateful for this gift and for all of the struggles that have led me to this place. It is from this humble place of knowing the fragility and vulnerability of being human and from the liberation that comes from healing, that I offer this book and my experience to you.

May your own liberation unfold in magical and beautiful ways.

Table of Contents

WIRED FOR HEALING:

Remapping the Brain to Recover from
Chronic and Mysterious Illnesses

Annie Hopper

CHAPTER I

My Story

In the summer of 2003 I moved to Kelowna, a medium-sized city in the interior of British Columbia, Canada. Shortly after I arrived there was a terrible forest fire that ravished the forest around the city and destroyed many homes on the periphery. Although I was lucky enough for the fire not to take my home as it had taken others' homes, there was thick smoke and falling ash every day for a couple of weeks. I didn't think much of it at the time except that I thought perhaps I should get the heck out of Dodge and move back to Vancouver. It was also during this period that I was in a seemingly minor motor vehicle accident, which resulted in cervical whiplash. This affected my central nervous system with the appearance of a Parkinson's like shake in my neck that lasted for months. A specialist diagnosed me at that time with a "dormant nervous tick" that was activated by the car accident. After months of rest and rehabilitation, I was unable to do things that would aggravate my neck in any way, but life moved forward and onward I went. By 2004, I was once again living a full and rewarding life as a successful counselor. My practice was fully booked with a waiting list. I had my own newspaper column called Emotional Rescue that was published weekly in the Kelowna Capital News. In my column, I advised readers on how to gain perspective and to navigate through life's emotional terrain. I was also featured as a regular guest on talk radio as an expert in emotional wellness. I was healthy, I was in a fulfilling relationship, I had lots of friends, I was involved in an amateur musical theatre group and a local choir and I felt connected to my community.

My counseling practice was booming and I moved into a new office. I painted it my favorite shade of green and bought all new furniture, hoping to create an inviting and sacred healing space. The irony of this hope would come to me later. What I didn't know was that there was mould in the building that I moved into, and that my brand new office space was formerly the janitor's supply room. I hadn't realized that my office lacked proper ventilation or that the new (smaller) janitor's supply room was now next door, sharing a wall.

Within a couple of months of working in my new office I slowly started to become sensitive to certain scented products. Perfumes and colognes had started to take on a stronger and more pungent smell that gave me headaches. I had also started to become sensitive to the washroom deodorizer that they used in the office building. I would often go home with headaches, muscle aches, and pains, and I was also experiencing frequent insomnia but was unaware of the cause. I tried to alleviate the symptoms in a number of different ways but they persisted.

In my former career as a registered massage therapist, I was very aware of the symbiotic connection between the mind and the body. Also, as a core belief counselor who was trained in emotional root cause analysis psychology, my first response to my own illness was to investigate the possibility of underlying emotional or psychological issues. Given my experience both personally and professionally with abuse and trauma, I was quite familiar with the unraveling process of trauma in the body and the emotional scarring. However, when I examined my life for possible emotional or psychological causes of my mysterious ailment, I found no lingering or unresolved trauma. Yet the symptoms continued.

My family doctor diagnosed my symptoms as fibromyalgia. At the time, this felt like a catch-all diagnosis, the kind doctors might come up with when they don't have an answer for you. He sent me for a CT scan to make sure I didn't have a tumor or something else that could explain my peculiar collection of symptoms, but the scan revealed nothing out of the ordinary. Over this time, I spent thousands of dollars on an endless list of both allopathic and alternative health care practices to no avail.

When I returned from a two-week holiday in September of 2005 I realized it was my office that was making me sick. The moment I walked back into the building it was like I was walking into a toxic wall. Because my sense of smell had heightened (a common symptom of chemical sensitivities), I could distinguish the smell of the mould that had been disguised by the bathroom deodorizer – and the combination of the two was startling. It was suddenly clear to me that the lethal combination of mould and chemicals was the illusive cause of my symptoms. My healing oasis had morphed into a toxic nightmare. In addition to the mould, the washroom deodorizer and the unventilated closet of cleaning chemicals next door, I was exposed to a high level of Volatile Organic Compounds (VOCs) from the new furniture, the carpets and the paint. Many VOCs like formaldehyde and other solvents, are neurotoxic and dangerous to human health and they also cause harm to the environment. My sense of smell was so acute that I was immediately able to detect all of the other thousands of chemicals in my day-to-day living environment! I knew they were contributing to the symptoms because I was suddenly experiencing them as a source of poison and imminent danger. Thus began the journey of seeking out safety through my sense of smell.

Looking back, I find it interesting that not one of the practitioners that I visited had inquired about my work or home environment as it related to chemical intolerance. Nor had they asked about chemical exposures such as recent renovations or about air quality, or other environmental conditions in my day-to-day spaces. Through my informal research, I estimate that chemical sensitivities are initially triggered by chemical exposure through home or office renovations in over 80% of sufferers.

Although the limbic system forms only a small part of our brain, it has a huge influence in how we live our lives. The limbic system interprets all of our sensory information which, in turn, decides how our bodies should respond to external stimuli. The limbic system is also involved in our response to stress, in our emotional responses to events around us, and in our involuntary protective mechanisms (like the 'fight-or-flight' response). It is particularly active when we are under stress or we are feeling anxious or threatened. The limbic system however, is also engaged symbiotically with the rest of the body and responds to our physical well being, our thoughts and our emotions. When the limbic system is not functioning properly, threat mechanisms can overfire and distort the interpretation of sensory information. Any form of accumulative stress can cause limbic system damage that leads to dysfunction and to neurological disorganization. Many forms of stress can affect this system, such as chemical, bacterial, viral, fungal, physical, psychological and emotional stress. Often it is a "perfect storm" of stressors that create limbic system disorganization (also known as cross wiring). This neural disorganization establishes involuntary trauma patterns in circuits of the brain that overactivate threat, protective and survival mechanisms. A number of conditions are associated with limbic system dysfunction and are, I believe, the result of an acquired brain injury.

This was the situation in which I found myself in April of 2006 when my symptoms of chemical sensitivity worsened and escalated rapidly. By this point neither my doctor nor any of the specialists I had seen were able to help me. It was a Friday night, the end of a long work week, and my partner, James, and I were looking forward to dining out at a local restaurant. After work I had stopped off at a bookstore and I happened to walk by a scented candle display. Within five minutes I could barely speak or focus. Light was painful, sound was painful and it felt like I had knives piercing through my head. It was like a bad migraine amped up one thousand times. The pain continued to get worse until it felt as if I was having some kind of brain hemorrhage. I decided not to go to the hospital, since they had been unable to help me before. The idea of going there seemed pointless and extremely painful. I went home, lay down in a darkened room with a cold cloth on my head and prayed for sleep.

When I awoke my entire world had changed. I woke up feeling like I was a different person in a different body, and I was now the star of my own personal horror film. I literally felt like I was being poisoned by everything around me. I could no longer wear my usual clothes because I was repulsed by the chemicals in the detergent residue, which had morphed into some kind of putrid and toxic smell. Chemicals in scented products, like any of my personal hygiene items and all of our household cleaning products, produced symptoms of headache, nausea, rapid heart rate, possible convulsions, difficulty breathing, cognitive impairment and loss of voice. This was followed by complete exhaustion, muscle pain and twitching, which could last for a number of days after any exposure.

It was my physical reactions to various stimuli that forced me to research the ingredients that were present in the products that I was reacting to – hoping that, by avoiding them, I might be able to stop the growing list of symptoms. What I discovered was that many of the chemicals found in everyday household products and textiles are neurotoxic and very harmful to our health. In fact, many chemicals found in popular products are known to be carcinogenic, however that has not stopped the manufacturing companies from producing them, nor has it stopped them from advertising these products as "good for you". The knowledge that I gained about chemicals in our environment and how to live a more healthy lifestyle is what I consider to be the gift of having experienced a limbic system injury. James and I changed all of our personal hygiene products and household cleaners to unscented, organic, vegetable based products.

Although this protected me from chemical exposure in my home, I knew I was still hypersensitive to any number of chemicals out in the world. I had become so sensitive to chemicals and fragrances that I had to insist that my clients only use organic and unscented personal hygiene products. I was very fortunate that they were compliant with my requests. In fact, they were more compliant than most of my friends at that time. However, even though they tried their best, accidents would happen. Perhaps they hugged someone before coming to see me who was wearing cologne or perfume. Or maybe they had a chemical deodorizer of some kind in their car. A minute amount of chemical residue on their clothing would be enough to send me into a tailspin of symptoms.

Eventually I could no longer work with my clients face to face. Being resourceful, I then offered telephone counseling. This worked for a while, but unfortunately the sensitivities worsened and multiplied. As the illness progressed, I needed less and less of an exposure to have a severe reaction, and the sensitivities were spreading to other sources like treated wood, textiles such as new clothes, and carpets, and paint (VOCs). I had gone from getting headaches and body aches for a few hours to having severe physical reactions, some life threatening, followed by extreme fatigue that would last for days.

As a result my life was becoming more and more isolated. I could no longer work, spend time with my friends, go to church, or be involved in any social outings. I am extremely grateful that James was compassionate and stayed with me through all of this. Although he did not fully understand what was happening, he did love me and supported me through it. I feel incredibly grateful for this as I realize now that, for many, this is not the case.

If my family or friends came to visit, they had to jump through the same hoops that my clients had had to. They too were given a personal hygiene list and if they did not adhere to this I wasn't willing or able to spend time with them. For some, there was also an element of disbelief about my illness and that doubt became another separating factor. The number of people that would actually come to our house to visit diminished because of the conditions that they had to meet beforehand. If someone arrived at the house and had accidentally picked up some kind of chemical residue, they knew they would have to shower and change into James's or my clothing for the duration of the visit. I would put their clothing in a plastic bag outside by the door. On leaving, I would go to the opposite end of the house while they would change and quickly leave. Needless to say, I was feeling increasingly isolated, lonely and depressed. My world was growing smaller and weirder by the day, and my hope for recovery was dwindling. Then just as I thought that things couldn't get worse…they did.

Looking back, I know now that I had suffered a brain injury, likely from a combination of mould and chemicals that affected the function of my limbic system. I know that my brain had gone into a self-protective cycle in response to the chemical injury. The brain circuits responsible for sensory perception and survival had cross wired in a brilliant attempt to protect me. However, this adaptive neuroplastic response had also created my living nightmare.

A year and a half after developing multiple chemical sensitivities my life became even more like a science fiction movie. Overnight I had become sensitive to electricity and I could no longer live in my own scent-free home. It was like a switch had gone off in my brain, and, all of a sudden, I could not only sense all electrical fields, but the electromagnetic fields were draining the energy from my body. I would lose my voice when I got close to any electricity and my body felt like it would go into convulsions at any moment. I could hear the piercingly high pitch tone of electricity and my head and my ears ached from the exposure. There was a metallic, electrical taste in my mouth – like shorted wires.

I walked around our condo, looking for a simple space where I was not affected by the electrical fields. I kept repeating the word hello as I walked, losing my voice every few feet from exposure to electrical fields. James looked at me with a worried and puzzled look on his face. The look said everything; he was wondering whether I had completely lost my mind. Yet he really knew I wasn't crazy. Yes, it was a crazy situation, but I was not crazy. He had seen what had happened to me with the chemical sensitivities and had found that condition difficult to accept in the beginning, too. He knew that I wasn't making this new sensitivity up and tried to reassure me that everything would be okay. I heard the words but they somehow seemed hollow when faced with the reality of not having anywhere to live.

All of a sudden my survival was the only thing that mattered. I was officially homeless. Not because I didn't have a home or I couldn't afford a home, but because my body could no longer tolerate living in that environment.

Camping became our temporary solution until I ended up living on a houseboat without heat and optional electricity. This was the only place I could find where I didn't react to environmental stressors like the chemical fragrances or electromagnetic fields that pervade everyone's living spaces constantly. When I could no longer tolerate living in my home I decided that I would do anything that I needed to in order to survive. This also meant that I had to move away from my partner, James. I lived in a rundown houseboat that was docked at the Comox Bay Marina, 12 hours away from my home. I spent five very lonely and depressing months there. At times, my will to live was thin. I was very grateful to have my dog Bella with me as a constant source of love and distraction from my suffering. James was also a constant source of support and would come to visit me every four weeks. This period of time was very difficult. I was very sick, depressed, lonely and scared and I was rapidly losing hope.

Environmental doctors and alternative health care practitioners alike view MCS largely as a toxic overload syndrome and the main treatments are detoxification, nutritional supplements and avoidance. Yet, even while I was undergoing detoxification treatments, I intuitively knew that a large part of my symptoms were due to a brain impairment.

I recognized that there was something missing from the medical models that guided my specialists' understandings of my condition. What if it wasn't just a toxic overload illness that required a detoxification regimen to undo it? What if the illness actually originated in the brain? What if the damage was also generated from the inside and not simply from the outside? The symptoms were so cognitive in nature that I just knew it had to be a neurological issue (brain injury) as opposed to a physical reaction like an allergy. I began to wonder why most people could walk down the laundry detergent aisle in a grocery store and not react like I did. This simple exposure would send me into a huge tailspin of symptoms for days. It was like my brain's "filtering system" just wasn't functioning properly and was affecting me on many different levels simultaneously; physically, emotionally and psychologically. I began to recognize a lot of the behavioural and emotional symptoms of a limbic system trauma pattern. This statement from my journal at the time kind of sums it up:

> "If I'm not careful the dark caverns of my mind are places that I can hide out in for days on end and that particular form of addiction just feeds on itself."

As a trained 'curious observer' I was able to look at my own illness and separate my own emotional baggage from the perceptual distortions caused by the trauma patterns. What I learned was that it wasn't particularly productive to keep analyzing the same negative emotions and thoughts, as one might in a behavioural psychology model. The negative emotion that would normally dissipate with attention and acknowledgement in a traditional therapeutic method, actually grow stronger in the case of a limbic system injury. The more attention you give to an established trauma pattern, the more rooted it becomes as a dysfunctional pathway in the brain. What I also recognized was that simply observing the thoughts or feelings was not enough. Observation skills created some distance, but this alone did not stop the trauma pattern.

As a core belief counselor I knew that a simple shift in my perspective and change in behaviour could change my reality. What I didn't know is whether it could change my physical reality in relation to my sensory perception.

Long before I ended up on the houseboat, I had begun to do

research on the human brain. I was looking for a correlation between the brain patterns or brain 'dysfunctions' across similar and overlapping illnesses such as chronic fatigue syndrome, fibromyalgia, post traumatic stress disorder, anxiety and depression. Much to my joy and validation, I found a series of articles and books that alluded to this and I knew I was headed in the right direction. Through my own experience and reading publications from leading researchers like Dr. Norman Doidge, Dr. Jeffery Schwartz, Dr. Bruce Lipton, Dr. Joe Dispenza, Dr. Jill Bolte Taylor and Dr. Candace Pert, I became familiar with the idea of neuroplasticity. (See list of articles of note in Appendix A).

My true introduction to neuroplasticity came by way of Dr. Norman Doidge's book, *The Brain That Changes Itself.* The term neuroplasticity refers to the brain's ability to change. It is an innate quality of the human brain and is neither positive nor negative; rather, it is reflective of our life experiences. The process of neuroplasticity is involved in all learning. It is how we learn to speak, to eat, and to tie our shoes. It is involved every time we learn a new fact, meet a new person, or see a new landscape. However, in response to trauma, the ways in which the brain changes are not always good or healthy. From Dr. Doidge, I learned about many different scientists in this field and the varied ways in which the human brain can structure and restructure itself, especially to accommodate any number of injuries, disabilities and seemingly incurable illnesses. Dr. Doidge's description of the plasticity of the brain gave me hope and renewed my determination to find a resolution to my own brain related illnesses. It inspired my "aha!" moment when I realized my illness could actually be a brain mechanism that was cross wired.

Once I started to entertain the idea that the threat and survival mechanisms in my brain were not functioning properly and that this malfunction could be at the root of illness, things began to change. However, it took me a full six months of rigorous practice to fully rewire my limbic system and return to living a "normal" and environmentally aware life.

What I realized is that MCS is more than just a toxic overload syndrome. The important piece in understanding this illness is that toxic exposure affects brain function and, more specifically, that it damages circuits within the limbic system of the brain. More importantly, what I discovered is that these disorganized neural circuits can be corrected.

The answer to diagnosing, treating and preventing limbic system injuries is multifaceted. One of the most important factors in treating limbic system conditions is to recognize that the root of the condition is located *physically* in the brain and is a form of an *acquired brain injury* that affects many systems of the body. These conditions are not psychological in nature, nor are the symptoms of a malfunctioning limbic system the products of self-delusion—they are real! Just like a nerve in another part of the body that can become injured, the brain can be injured by a variety of traumas: viruses (such as mononucleosis), bacteria (such as the one that causes Lyme disease), head and neck injuries, chemical exposure, mould, emotional or psychological trauma (such as witnessing the horrors of war), or any combination of these. Therefore, just as one would go to a physiotherapist for rehabilitation of, say, a muscle injury, so the Dynamic Neural Retraining System™ (DNRS) that I developed is designed to rehabilitate the limbic system.

CHAPTER 2

The Limbic System: an Overview

To begin, let me say that I am not a neuroscientist or a doctor, and that the following explanation is *my* understanding of the limbic system. Depending on your source, information about the limbic system may vary. What I am trying to convey in this chapter is my best understanding of how trauma can affect the survival centres of the brain in the limbic system, and how this relates to illness in the body.

This chapter describes the structure and function of the limbic system, and as such, it can be a bit demanding to read, especially if you are having troubles with concentration or with memory. Don't worry if you can't get through it easily or if you can't remember the details, but at least give it a try. It's helpful to have an understanding of how limbic injury affects health.

The limbic system is a collection of brain structures located in the mid brain that is typically known as 'the emotional brain.' It was formerly known as the *rhinencephalon*, derived from Greek roots which literally mean 'smell brain.' Our sense of smell is the only sense that actually bypasses other filtering stations in the brain.

The limbic system is comprised of the amygdala, the hippo-campus, the cingulate cortex, and the hypothalamus. The limbic system is the part of the brain that is responsible for interpreting, categorizing, and sorting sensory input. It filters the billion bits of information that we experience at any given moment, and it determines how we code, remember, and respond to them. It stores memories, regulates hormones, and is also involved in motor function. The limbic system is a large part of our primitive defense mechanism.

The limbic system also regulates function of the parasympathetic and sympathetic nervous systems, which means it regulates things like pulse, blood pressure, breathing, and arousal in response to emotional circumstances. It plays an important role in friendship, bonding, love, affection, and the expression of mood. The limbic system is the 'first responder' in every situation to both perceived and real threats, sending cascading messages to the rest of the body to react accordingly. It serves as a protective gate to analyze and filter incoming stimuli and assigns a level of importance to each potential threat.

The brain works by patterns of association – it automatically sorts incoming stimuli into patterns that it already recognizes. We learn through experience what produces pain, pleasure, danger, and fear. For instance, when we put our hand on a hot stove, it only takes one experience for us to learn that this action results in pain. Equally we only need to taste sugar once in order to want that pleasure again. For basic survival purposes, the brain generalizes information about our environment to minimize potential danger. This is thought to be an involuntary and unconscious process. Under normal circumstances, the protective mechanism of the limbic system would only become activated in times of danger or threat. However, if the limbic system is impaired, it will adapt itself in response to the injury and can cause cross wiring or disorganization of 'normal' neuronal circuits in the brain. This, in turn, can cause distorted unconscious reactions, sensory perceptions, and protective responses.

When limbic system function is impaired, it can alter the way that your brain and body interprets, encodes, and responds to any sensory stimuli. Over time this pattern of distorted perception and reaction becomes habitual and can result in a range of neurological, immunological, and endocrine system abnormalities. Physical, mental, and emotional traumas have the ability to alter limbic system function and can damage any number of neurons along this cascading system. Damage to the limbic system can severely alter the interpretation of incoming sensory information and, in turn, alter our ability to inhibit our physiological and behavioral reactions.

THE AMYGDALA

The amygdala is typically known as the fear center of the brain. In fact, all emotion is processed by the amygdala, but it is particularly good at monitoring our environment for danger. The amygdala is involved in both emotional learning and memory, as it responds strongly to all emotional stimuli, but especially to fear. Studies show that the amygdala along with the insula and the anterior cingulate cortex constitute the 'fear network' of the brain (Holzschneider, K., Mulert, C., 2011). The amygdala is also associated with negative emotions like anger and rage. It enhances the emotional aspects of a memory, allowing it to be processed at a deeper level and accessed more quickly for faster response. This is an ancient unconscious protective mechanism. When the amygdala senses danger, it sends direct messages to the body in a language that the body recognizes – stress hormones. In an extreme case, activation of the amygdala can trigger automatic body movements like jumping back, running away, or pulling someone out of danger. Any stimulus that has been categorized through experience as dangerous bypasses the sensory cortex of the brain and immediately activates the amygdala. In other words, the brain automatically reacts to the stimulus before we become consciously aware of it. Our emotional state will also dictate how an experience is remembered. Research has shown that the greater the intensity of emotion associated with the event, the higher the chance it will be remembered.

THE HIPPOCAMPUS

Due to its seahorse-like shape, the name *hippocampus* stems from the term 'seahorse' after the Greek *hippos* 'horse' and *kampos* 'sea monster.'

The hippocampus is involved in the process known as 'memory consolidation' which is the process of converting information from short-term to long-term memory. It assigns meaning and value to incoming information and is responsible for storing and retrieving long-term memories. It is important in forming new memories and connecting our emotions to our senses, such as smell and sound, to memories. Damage to this area of the brain may result in an inability to provide a safe context for incoming information. Changes in hippocampal function can also affect the ability to form new memories.

Jill Bolte Taylor put this very succinctly in her book *My Stroke of Insight* (2006):

> *The primary job of the amygdala is to scan all incoming stimulation in this immediate moment and determine the level of safety. One of the jobs of the cingulate gyrus of the limbic system is to focus the brain's attention.*
>
> *When incoming stimulation is perceived as familiar, the amygdala is calm and the adjacently positioned hippo-*

campus is capable of learning and memorizing new information. However, as soon as the amygdala is triggered by unfamiliar or perhaps threatening stimulation, it raises the brain's level of anxiety and focuses the mind's attention on the immediate situation. Under these circumstances, our attention is shifted away from the hippocampus and focused toward self-preserving behavior about the present moment.

Sensory information streams in through our sensory systems and is immediately processed through our limbic system. By the time a message reaches our cerebral cortex for higher thinking, we have already placed a "feeling" upon how we view that stimulation – is this pain or is this pleasure? Although many of us may think of ourselves as thinking creatures that feel, biologically we are feeling creatures that think.

CINGULATE CORTEX

The cingulate cortex is involved with autonomic functions such as regulating heart rate, blood pressure, and cognitive and attentional processing. The anterior cingulate cortex (ACC) receives sensory inputs from the thalamus and sends outputs to several brain regions such as the hippocampus and amygdala. The ACC provides a pathway from the thalamus to the hippocampus, focuses attention on emotionally significant events, and associates memories to smells and to pain.

The cingulate cortex is involved in memory, emotional processing, and learning. The anterior cingulate cortex is activated by intense emotion (both positive and negative) and relays this information to the amygdala. Activation of the ACC increases during intense emotions like love, anger, or lust. It is also involved in processing pain and perceived pain and is the place in the brain where pain and emotion meet.

The ACC is particularly active in tasks that demand judgment and discrimination. The ACC is involved in the establishment and consolidation of different forms of memory associated with fear. The anterior cingulate gyrus is primarily involved in signaling the presence of conflict and/or error. Overactivation of the ACC is associated with an increase in startle response and harm avoidance behaviours (Shum,F.W, Wu, Lo, Zhao, M. Yoyoda, H., Xu, H, Ren, M., Ren, M. Pinaud, R. Ko, S., Lee, Y. Daang, B., Zhou, M., 2007). Injury and inflammation can cause sensitivity in the ACC, affecting its ability to filter incoming information in a healthy way which can lead to to an extreme increase in the activation of fear networks.

In relation to limbic system conditions, the particularly interesting function of the cingulate cortex is that it mediates the response to noxious stimuli. When not functioning properly, the ACC can cause an 'over-focus' on the intensity of both perceived and real threats. In this case, it acts as a guard at the gateway of the brain, sending alarm messages to the rest of the brain. Damage to any cells along this neural network could considerably change the function of the cingulate cortex, thereby altering its function and its perception of harm, and contributing to the chronic stress response that is implicated in many illnesses.

HYPOTHALAMUS

The hypothalamus is said to be 'the brain of the brain.' It is connected to many parts of the central nervous system. It is the control center of all autonomic regulatory activities of the body. It is like having an internal chemist as it produces powerful brain hormones which relay information and instructions to all parts of the brain and body. It is responsible for maintaining homeostasis in the body through the cardiovascular system, temperature regulation, and abdominal visceral regulation. It manages endocrine hormonal levels, sensory processing, body metabolism, and eating and drinking behaviours.

The hypothalamus is principally involved in the mind/body connection. It links the nervous system to the endocrine system via the pituitary gland. The hypothalamus integrates all of the five senses, namely taste, smell, sight, sound, and touch, then translates, distills, and assembles the information into one distinct 'package,' combining all the attributes of an experience, along with all the associated stimuli, into one simple conceptual unit. When an entire series of neural networks are activated in any given moment of time, the brain then releases a specific neural cocktail that represents that moment, and collectively they represent a specific feeling. The brain then stores this sequence of neural activation as an emotional memory, complete with an understanding of and an evaluation of the experience.

The limbic system's intricate makeup is increasingly vulnerable to injury as a result of trauma from the higher incidence of stressors in our environment than were present in the past. Accumulative trauma can also have an affect on limbic system function, thereby making it more susceptible to injury. Damage to any area or to any structure within the limbic system can result in distorted perception, evaluation, and response to stimuli. These altered responses happen on an unconscious, physiological level and can contribute to emotional, psychological, and physical symptoms in sufferers of any number of limbic system related conditions. While limbic system dysfunction is involved in many chronic and mysterious illnesses, the following chapter provides an overview of some of the most common conditions.

CHAPTER 3

How to Identify a Limbic System Impairment

Damage to the limbic system is commonly caused by a toxic injury. A patient's symptoms may seem vague and unrelated; however, neurotoxicity – poisoning of the brain and nervous system – can affect *all* systems of the body and lead to multi-organ, and multi-system malfunction. This makes sense when we realize the brain and nervous system control all bodily functions. While physical symptoms may be the most apparent, the fact must be considered that the patient has most likely suffered toxic injury and has likely sustained damage to the brain and nervous system as a result. One must also understand that neurotoxicity is not widely documented. For example, the damage sustained from a toxic injury may not necessarily affect brain structure at levels that are visible through a magnetic resonance imaging (MRI) or a computerized tomography (CT) scan. Most neurologists are not trained in toxicology, nor are they taught that common chemicals in our environment can cause toxic trauma to the brain and body. Therefore, they may not be aware that a patient's symptoms are related to a toxic brain injury. In fact, patients who suggest that symptoms were caused or exacerbated by a chemical exposure may encounter denial or resistance on the part of medical professionals, or they may simply be diagnosed as 'malingering.'

Neurotoxic trauma can affect the patients' ability to think, to control emotions, to perceive, to plan, to work, to manage their lives, or to move freely through the world around them. In severe cases, the injury can cause the patient to become completely disabled, severely affecting their quality of life and their ability to participate in normal society.

Limbic system impairment is often elusive and difficult to diagnose using traditional methods. Many symptoms are mistakenly thought to be attributed to other illnesses, but they do not respond successfully to traditional treatments. A limbic system impairment is psychoneuroimmunological (PNI) in nature, which means it involves psychological processes as well as the nervous and immune systems of the body. Consequently, a limbic system impairment expresses itself via the central nervous system, which can affect our state of physical, psychological, and/or emotional health. Impairment may be caused from physical injury (head or neck trauma), toxicant injury from chemicals, electromagnetic fields/radiation, bacteria, viruses, fungi, exposure to moulds and/or psychological or emotional stress. All of these can result in brain trauma, inducing overactivation of the mechanisms within the deep limbic system circuits in the brain that deal with threat, with self-protection, and with survival, and they can initiate a multiple system breakdown in the body. Or to put it another way, the brain gets 'stuck' in an unconscious state of chronic emergency that perpetuates illness and inflammation. This typically involves the central nervous system, the musculoskeletal system, the respiratory system, the immune system, the digestive system, and the endocrine system. No wonder the symptoms seem unrelated, even to medical professionals!

Often there is a trigger that precedes the onset of illness such as a renovation to one's office or home, pesticide exposure or other kinds of chemical exposure, a head or neck injury, a viral or bacterial infection, mould or fungus exposure, a reaction to prescribed medication, surgery, and/or extreme psychological or emotional trauma (e.g. loss of a loved one, divorce, moving, etc.).

With this in mind, the following list of questions will help to identify a limbic system impairment.

QUESTIONAIRE

Do you suffer from 'brain fog' or unexplained headaches?

Do you suffer from low energy?

Do you suffer from chronic joint and/or muscle pain?

Do you find yourself constantly 'body checking' for symptoms of pain or discomfort?

Do you have a heightened sense of smell or taste?

Do you have other heightened sensory perceptions, such as light, sound or electromagnetic sensitivities?

Do perfumes or other chemical products (e.g. household cleaners, personal hygiene products, paint, adhesives, new textiles or carpets, etc.) give you headaches or make you feel nauseous or lightheaded?

Do you get noticeably irritable, anxious, or upset when around specific scents?

Have you had your home, office, or other space renovated recently?

Do you suffer from anxiety or panic attacks?

Do you purposely avoid going to specific places or doing specific things because of your health condition or because of the potential health risks?

Do you have sleep-related issues?

Are you limited in what you can do physically due to your health issues?

Do you have a number of food sensitivities?

Are you unable to take prescribed medications?

Have your health conditions affected your job?

Have your health conditions affected your relationships with your friends and family?

Do you have problems accessing medical care due to your sensitivities?

Have you been to see a number of practitioners that were unable to diagnosis your condition or effectively treat it?

Do you experience pronounced mood swings?

Do you find it difficult to focus or concentrate?

Do you dwell on past negative events?

Do you find yourself expecting negative outcomes?

Do you have short-term memory problems?

Do you worry a lot?

Do you often feel depressed?

Do you still experience symptoms of illness despite the fact that you live in a healthy home?

Have you tried detoxification treatments and nutritional supplements yet still find that you are symptomatic?

If you answered 'yes' to more than 5 of these questions, it is likely that you are experiencing a limbic system impairment. If this is the case, you would likely benefit from 'rewiring' your limbic system.

LIMBIC SYSTEM DYSFUNCTION AND RELATED CONDITIONS

The limbic system is influenced by a number of stimuli, any of which may cause it to have an associative survival response. Emotional, physical, psychological, chemical, viral, fungal, and bacterial trauma can all influence limbic system function. Some examples of trauma that activate the threat mechanism in the brain are heavy metal toxicity or chemical exposure, excessive electromagnetic radiation, medications, head or neck injury, physical pain, inflammation, surgery, psychological stress, accumulated stress, emotional trauma, viruses, bacterial or fungal infections, or exposure to mould. Often it is a combination of multiple stressors that create a 'perfect storm' that triggers limbic system dysfunction.

When the limbic system is impaired, it naturally adapts itself in response to injury. The resulting cross wiring establishes involuntary trauma patterns in neural circuits of the brain that can cause overactivation of threat, protective, and survival mechanisms. The hyperactivated threat mechanisms can alter perception of stimuli and send impending danger and survival messages to all other systems of the body.

This innate adaptive response is known as neuroplasticity. However, the ways in which the brain can change in response to trauma or damage are not always good or healthy (Hermans, Erno J., et al, 2011).

An initial limbic system injury is followed by an inflammatory and chronic stress response that moves the brain and body from a state of growth and repair into a state of chronic crisis or emergency. This affects our energy production, ability to fight disease, rest and digestion processes, pain perception, cognitive function, and emotional state. It can also increase inflammatory responses and alter sensory perception, including smell, taste, light, sound, touch, and energetic senses, that is, sensations that generate from within the body or what we sense external to the body.

The brain is directly wired to the immune system so it comes as no surprise that limbic system impairment and a chronic 'fight-or-flight' state would affect the ability to fight disease. Chronic stress can also lead to damaging levels of inflammation. Additionally, studies have suggested that chronic stress can reactivate latent viruses as well as change gene expression (Merchang, J., 2013), (Kiecolt-Glaser, J. K., Speicher, C. E., Holliday, J. E., Glaser, R., 1984), (Cole, S. W., Hawkley, L. C., Arevalo, J. M., Sung, C. Y., Rose, R. M., Cacioppo, J. T., 2007).

With regard to chemical, electrical, and other environmental sensitivities, after the initial damage to the brain, the 'fight-or-flight' centres become overactivated to toxicants in the environment, causing sufferers to have heightened sensory perception and react to toxicants at levels far below what people normally react to. When threat mechanisms in the limbic system are overactivated, it leads to faulty integration of sensory information. For instance, according to a 2012 study (Krusemark, E. A. and Li, W., 2012), general anxiety causes an increase in amygdala and hippocampus activity and a heightened sense of smell in relation to perceived threat (negative odour). An individual may be completely unaware of specific sensory perceptions until the limbic system is injured and perception is heightened to an extreme level, such as with an abnormal ability to perceive chemicals or electromagnetic fields.

Chemical sensitivities, fibromyalgia, chronic fatigue syndrome and electric hypersensitivity syndrome are all characterized as toxicant induced loss of tolerance, or TILT-associated illnesses (Miller, 1997). A toxicant injury to the brain, caused by chemicals, bacteria, viruses, electromagnetic fields, and/or psychological or emotional stress can cause a neuroimmunological response, that is, a response which affects brain and immune system function. Symptoms of these conditions can manifest themselves on physical, psychological, and emotional levels.

Patients are often misdiagnosed with a psychiatric disorder due to the extreme nature and scope of symptoms. Understandably, anyone who is suffering from a chronic illness and the devastating affects on their quality of life will undoubtedly also be affected by their experience of extreme stress. It is not uncommon for patients to develop psychological conditions over the course of their illness. However, many conditions such as anxiety and depression are often associative and are not at the root of the illness as is sometimes assumed.

Overactivation of threat centres in the limbic system are related to survival emotions including fear, rage, anger, worry, depression, hopelessness, and catastrophic thinking. According to Singer and Johnson (2006), "More than 850 industrial and commercial chemicals are known to cause neurobehavioral disorders." These symptoms can be present to varying degrees in all limbic system related conditions and are not limited to chemical sensitivities.

Physiological reactions to exposure or perceived threat can include severe mood swings, sudden and severe depression, rage, crying, and suicidal ideation (preoccupation with thoughts of suicide). Patients are often emotionally overreactive to stress, which can exaggerate physical symptoms. Some cannot cry with appropriate stimulus, e.g. even with the death of a loved one. In contrast, others are unable to genuinely laugh. Patients also have a general difficulty accessing positive emotional states or positive memories. They often have an exaggerated startle response and extreme harm avoidance behaviours. In addition to the emotional symptoms, patients may also experience psychological symptoms such as hyper vigilance, a heightened sense of threat, negative self-absorption, and a tendency toward blame and defensiveness.

When fear centres in the brain become chronically activated, it can feel as though your brain has been hijacked. Amygdala hijack is defined by Wikipedia as follows:

> *Amygdala hijack is a term coined by Daniel Goleman in his 1996 book Emotional Intelligence: Why It Can Matter More Than IQ (1996). Drawing on the work of Joseph E. LeDoux (1996), Goleman uses the term to describe emotional responses from people which are immediate and*

overwhelming, and out of measure with the actual stimu-
lus because it has triggered a much more significant emo-
tional threat.

Stimulus from the thalamus goes to both the amygdala (the emotional brain) and the neocortex (the thinking brain). However, if the stimulus is a categorical match with a prior threat association, information travels faster to the amygdala and overrides the neocortex. In other words, threat messages are received faster and take priority, which can lead to reactions that may be inappropriate to the stimulus.

When the threat centres are activated by trauma, the amygdala triggers a 'fight-or-flight' response and sends alarm messages to the hypothalamus (the relay station in the brain) that then sends messages to the adrenal glands (near the kidneys) to release adrenaline into the bloodstream. When a stress response is chronic, it releases a constant stream of stress hormones into the body that can further damage the brain.

Overactivation of threat, survival, and protective mechanisms can also lead to hyperactivity within the amygdala and a misinterpretation of threat-related stimuli. The anterior cingulate cortex becomes overly focused on the threat potential of stimuli. The inadequate function of the anterior cingulate cortex adapts to this dysfunction, resulting in the inaccurate evaluation of other stimuli as potential threat. This, in turn, influences hippocampal function in its explicit memory capability and its ability to identify safe contexts. This response to stimuli is not processed at a conscious level.

There is strong evidence that the amygdala can trigger a full-scale threat response without conscious awareness of threat related stimulus (Gilbert, B., 2010). Commonly, limbic system conditions are characterized by amygdala hyperactivity, anterior cingulate deficiency, hippocampal deficiency, and a heightened stress response.

This cascading stress response can trigger the hypothalamus to release specific neurotransmitters that may keep the brain and body in a chronic state of stress which, in turn, can negatively affect multiple systems.

In a limbic system trauma loop, the hypothalamus releases stress hormones, the amygdala is activated in a fear/protective response, the cingulate cortex focuses the brain on the perceived threat, and the hippocampus keeps track of the experience for future reference and protection.

Anatomical connections between the amygdala, hippocampus, and hypothalamus facilitate the activation of the limbic-hypothalamic-pituitary-adrenal axis or HPA axis. Sensory information arriving in the amygdala is processed and conveyed to several parts of the brain involved with responses to fear. Overactivation of the threat mechanisms cause a chronic stress response resulting in HPA hyper-reactivity. The HPA axis controls reactions to stress and regulates many body processes, including digestion, the immune system, mood and emotions, sexual arousal, and the storage and expenditure of energy. Chronic activation of the HPA axis causes increased production of stress hormones that perpetuate a negative feedback loop. As the brain is constantly taking cues from the body, the chronic release of stress hormones keeps the brain in a 'fight-or-flight' state. This adaptive response to trauma is referred to as a limbic system trauma loop.

Over time, the chronic activation of the threat response becomes automatically wired in the brain. This speaks to Canadian psychologist Donald Hebb's great contribution to the understanding of neuroplasticity: "neurons that fire together – wire together" (1949). Basically this means that neurons that coactivate at any given time will do so automatically with repetition. This is at the foundation of all learning. But in the case of a limbic system trauma, this is also at the root of much suffering. The sensitivities that develop through the reinforcement of the trauma loop can also spread to other forms of sensory stimulation.

A process of sensitization, called 'kindling,' often occurs where sufferers will find themselves reacting to lesser amounts of stimuli and more classes of chemical substances (e.g., synthetic fragrances, smoke, pesticides, etc.) and may even progress to natural or inert substances by unconscious association (flowers, essential oils, or food smells). The sensitivities can also spread to other forms of sensory stimulation such as touch, hearing, sight (light sensitivity), and food.

With a compromised limbic system, the threat mechanisms of the brain are constantly on high alert and with specific exposures, are launched into an extreme aversion reaction. A minute amount of stimuli can throw the whole system into a five–alarm stress response. Because the threat mechanism is triggered by toxicants in the environment, the patient will naturally learn to avoid triggers in a protective response. While we understand that environmental toxins can be the cause of limbic system injury, it is important to note that the injury itself can cause altered sensory perception and lead to a negative feedback loop.

Once in survival mode, the limbic system reacts by physically focusing the body's energy on survival. Energy is taken away from other mechanisms associated with growth and regeneration, like communication between cells, absorption of nutrients, production of energy, excretion of waste products, or rest. Research has shown that chronic or excessive stress inhibits synaptic function and neuronal growth.

This trauma cycle keeps the individual in a state of physiological 'emergency' that involves the central nervous system and the musculoskeletal system as well as the respiratory, gastro-intestinal, immunological, and endocrine systems, causing a range of physical symptoms that are often disabling. It can also keep the individual in a state of hyper-vigilance and focused on personal health and safety. The combination of the compromised functioning of the body's systems along with the symptomatic hyper-focus on health and protection can leave the patient in a state of physical, emotional, and psychological crisis.

In a nutshell, this means that the brain and body unconsciously get stuck in a permanent 'fight-or-flight' response. In this emergency state, the brain perceives a constant threat akin to being hunted by a ferocious tiger, even if there is no tiger. When suffering from a limbic system injury, the brain can be sending the body false messages about threat perception, pain, and distorted sensory perception.

It is thought that the pathogenesis of limbic system dysfunction that is associated with many chronic illnesses is caused from trauma to the brain that affects self-protective mechanisms which overactivates fear centres of the brain that leads to a chronic stress response. Over time, chronic overactivation of the fear centres in the brain can structurally change the brain and thus its function. This can also lead to altered sensory function and perception. In some ways, these illnesses are much like post-traumatic stress disorder (PTSD). With PTSD, the memory of a trauma does not shift into the past; rather, the person relives the trauma on a daily basis because their brain is stuck in a trauma pattern.

There is considerable overlap between PTSD and many other limbic system-related illnesses like multiple chemical sensitivities, chronic fatigue syndrome, fibromyalgia and electric hypersensitivity syndrome. With PTSD, the involved trauma is most often triggered by a severe psychological event. The brain is so overwhelmed at the time that it does not have the capacity to file the event into the past, causing a disorganization of neural networks during an extreme stress situation (Rauch, S. L., Shin, L.M., Wright, C., 2003). Many other limbic system conditions are similar in nature to PTSD in that during the initial trauma, the brain cannot filter the incoming information and gets stuck in a trauma cycle. This can affect perception and the ability to evaluate incoming sensory information. Some people are more susceptible to this type of injury given their genetic makeup, which can alter detoxification pathways. However, whether the gene is present or not, the limbic system can still be rewired.

QUALITY OF LIFE

Above and beyond personal health considerations, people that suffer from many of these conditions are also faced with a number of practical concerns and challenges such as the difficulty in finding environmentally compatible housing, the lack of recognition of these conditions, accurate diagnosis and appropriate treatment from the medical industry, financial strain, social isolation, and lack of emotional support. Many are unable to access basic healthcare such as seeing dentists or doctors due to physical limitations associated with the illness. All of these factors combine to perpetuate an emotional and psychological state of extreme stress.

Normally high-functioning and healthy individuals become shadows of their former selves. These conditions literally rob them of their ability to function in the world. Some lose their jobs and their homes, and in severe cases live in extreme isolation and pain. Most cannot travel and often become housebound, and some even become homeless.

The amount of suffering that people endure as a result of toxic injury and impaired limbic system function can be extreme and devastating for both the sufferer and their families. Loved ones often do not understand the condition and may come to view the patient as high maintenance, controlling, or just plain crazy. Many patients fall into a life of extraordinary isolation, pain, and suffering.

Understandably, when suffering from a limbic system condition, the patient's predominant thought patterns are focused on how to avoid further suffering. The majority of thought processes are concerned with preservation of health and avoidance of illness. This way of thinking acts as a protective mechanism to ensure that the patient's already compromised state of health does not deteriorate further. While the body's response to the tiniest amount of chemical or electromagnetic fields may seem overreactive, it is not an emotional ploy, a control tactic, an allergy, or a psychological 'issue.' The body's actual response is a physical reality, and at times these reactions may, in fact, be life-threatening.

Given this state of constant stress, it is easy to understand the resultant patterns of negative thinking and feeling. However, it is important to keep in mind that such repetitive patterns promote specific neural network firing sequences, which take a distinct pathway in the brain. The more travelled the pathway, the faster the firing sequences happen. The thought and emotional patterns involved are situational, but more importantly they are a symptom of limbic system dysfunction. For example, if patients' reactions are not being triggered by stimuli in their immediate situation, they may unconsciously ponder old trauma or ruminate on past experiences of trauma.

The rational or consequential feelings that are associated with a limbic system trauma are predominately fear and worry.

The patient may also feel depressed, helpless, hopeless, angry, resentful, or even suicidal. In addition, because the filtering system in the 'emotional brain' isn't working properly, a patient may have uncontrollable 'emotional' reactions to toxicant stimuli. But what is normally interpreted as an emotional reaction may now express itself as a strictly physiological reaction to stimuli, such as spontaneous crying or inappropriate fits of rage.

This is not to say that concerns about the toxic elements of the environment are not rational. A toxic environment, without doubt, negatively impacts the brain and body. Nor does this mean that the emotional symptoms of limbic system impairment are strictly psychological in nature. Rather, in a more inclusive understanding of these conditions, the perception of threat (chemical or otherwise) and emotional reactions to threat have been altered by a physical brain injury. Understanding that these reactions are symptoms of the condition can alleviate further stress and help sufferers in the recovery process.

Most people suffering from a limbic system impairment will naturally try to avoid further exposure to whatever triggers symptoms of illness. Protective behaviours are justified when the consequence of not protecting oneself leads to further suffering. This makes sense when a person has no other method to cope with the symptoms, and at first this avoidance will result in the decrease of symptoms. However, long-term protective behaviours actually feed the threat mechanism. The more a patient reacts with fear to a certain stimulus, the stronger the association to that stimulus. The stronger the association, the faster the patient will react. With repetition, the pattern is ingrained, and the reaction becomes an unconscious process. Indeed, the patient's body may even react without conscious awareness of the stimuli.

LIMBIC SYSTEM CONDITIONS

Limbic system conditions are a relatively new occurrence (i.e. since WW ll). Today millions of people are affected with limbic system conditions worldwide and are rarely diagnosed appropriately, as many in the medical profession have yet to familiarize themselves with the affects of acquired toxic brain trauma and neuroplasticity-based treatments. Although different conditions will manifest a large variety of symptoms (some symptoms may overlap) and may have quite distinct causes, it is important to note that these conditions are all associated with limbic system injury and are greatly affected by limbic system reorganization. Fortunately, the Dynamic Neural Retraining System™ (DNRS) can be applied to a wider range of conditions, such as post-traumatic stress disorder, chronic pain, food sensitivities, depression, obsessive compulsive disorder, anxiety related disorders, postural orthostatic tachycardia syndrome, irritable bowel syndrome, Gulf War syndrome (GWS), and a host of other inflammatory conditions but, for the purposes of this book, I have focused on the following conditions; multiple chemical sensitivities, chronic fatigue syndrome, fibromyalgia, and electric hypersensitivity syndrome.

MYSTERIOUS CHRONIC ILLNESSES – HOW PREVALENT ARE THEY?

Millions suffer from chronic and mysterious illnesses triggered by everyday environmental toxins. Many people are misdiagnosed, while others are simply unaware that they are suffering from a toxic brain trauma or that neuro-rehabilitation is possible.

In 2005, according to Statistics Canada's Canadian Community Health survey, 1,135,000 Canadians had been diagnosed with one or more of ES/MCS (environmental sensitivities/multiple chemical sensitivities), myalgic encephalomyelitis/ chronic fatigue syndrome (ME/CFS) and/or fibromyalgia (FM). By 2010, this number increased to 1,415,000. Though Canada's population grew by only 7%, these conditions increased by an average of 25%. The current total population of Canada is approximately 35 million, whereas the United States population is approximately 317 million. If the rates of occurrence for these conditions in Canada are comparable to the U.S., then it would be reasonable to estimate at least 13 million people in the U.S. currently suffer from the conditions of MCS, CFS, and FM. It is also reasonable to assume this number stands to grow due to the increasing trend of these illnesses. These numbers will also rise due to the medical industry's growing awareness and the technical and scientific advancements that are improving physicians' ability to diagnose these conditions.

An example of this is the case of chemical sensitivities, where patients are either mildly or severely affected by common chemicals found in everyday living. For some, the symptoms could be mild like getting a headache after smelling perfume, while others may have more extreme reactions; for example, they may go into seizures from exposure to low levels of chemicals found in cleaning products. Fortunately, awareness of chemical sensitivity is growing along with its prevalence. For example, the California State Department of Health Services conducted a population-based survey in 1999 suggesting 85,000 new cases of chemical sensitivity per year in California.

However, the latest research by Dr. Claudia Miller now suggests 22% of individuals with chronic health issues suffer from some degree of chemical intolerance. Dr. Miller is an environmental health expert at the University of Texas School of Medicine in San Antonio whose expertise was recognized in the November 2013 feature article of *Discover Magazine* entitled

"Extreme Chemical Sensitivity Makes Sufferers Allergic to Life" (Neimark, J. 2013). *The article's subtitle* provides a comprehensive synopsis of the issue: "Its sufferers were once dismissed as hypochondriacs, but there's growing biological evidence to explain toxicant-induced loss of tolerance (TILT)." The article continues:

> *TILT, says (Dr. Claudia) Miller, is a two step process: First, a susceptible individual gets sick after toxic exposure or exposures. But then, instead of recovering, the neurological and immune systems remain damaged, and the individual fails to get well. The sufferer begins to lose tolerance to a wide range of chemicals common in everyday life. The latest research, both in the United States and abroad, suggest that brain processing itself is altered so that the neurological set point for sensitivity falls. The person, now sick, becomes highly sensitive to chemical exposures.*

Dr. Miller developed the *Quick Environment Exposure and Sensitivity Inventory* (QEESI) to create awareness of these illnesses and to help doctors diagnose their patients. Validated in Sweden, Denmark, Japan, and the United States, the QEESI is the most widely used screening instrument for chemical intolerance. The survey measures variables such as degree of chemical intolerance, symptom severity, and impact on life.

Many of these chronic and mysterious conditions are caused by toxins in our environment; however, even those within the medical system who are aware of toxic overload are not aware of how common everyday toxins affect brain function or how to rewire the brain for optimal health.

MULTIPLE CHEMICAL SENSITIVITIES (MCS)

MCS is also known as environmental illness, toxic injury, chemical sensitivity, chemical injury syndrome, 20th-century syndrome, sick building syndrome, idiopathic environmental intolerance, or toxicant-induced loss of tolerance (TILT). This is a disorder in which a person develops symptoms from exposure to chemicals in the environment. With each incidence of exposure, lower levels of the chemical will trigger a reaction, and the person becomes increasingly vulnerable to reactions triggered by chemicals.

In some cases, MCS is triggered by a single high-dose chemical exposure such as pesticide exposure or, quite commonly, chemical exposure from materials in a new home or in home renovations. For other patients, symptoms set in gradually from long-term chemical exposure or consistent low-grade chemical use, such as occurs when someone is residing or working in a poorly ventilated building, or when someone makes regular use of chemically based cosmetics or cleaning products. MCS is often seen in war veterans, specifically from the Gulf War (GWS) where there was a high incidence of exposure to chemicals in pesticides, smoke and gases, and vaccinations, all combined with a high degree of psychological stress.

Common symptoms of MCS include a heightened sense of smell/taste of chemicals, loss of voice with exposure, irregular heartbeat, headaches and/or migraines, extreme fatigue, muscle and/or joint pain, insomnia, asthma, sinus problems, eczema, rashes, nausea and vomiting, intestinal problems, seizures, short-term memory loss, difficulty concentrating, brain fog, irritability, mood swings, feelings of hopelessness, depression, anxiety, and isolation and avoidance behaviours.

MCS physically changes a patient's sensory perception. As

a result, perfumes and other scented products are experienced as toxic and potentially lethal chemical exposures. Chemicals in scented products begin to take on a toxic, sharp, and pungent quality that is akin to smelling a poisonous bug spray, and the brain reacts to the stimulus as it would to lethal poison. Depending on the severity of the condition, even the tiniest amount can be perceived as life-threatening because a patient who suffers from limbic system trauma has a heightened and altered perception of the intensity of the threat.

Triggers include perfumes and other fragrances, household cleaning products, detergents, formaldehyde, pesticides, solvents, petrochemical fuels such as diesel, gasoline, and kerosene, waxes, plastics, synthetic materials, treated wood products, tobacco smoke, mould, artificial colors, flavours, preservatives, and volatile organic compounds often found in paint, new textiles, furniture, and carpeting.

This could be due to damage caused by frequent exposure to more than 100,000 chemicals in the products commonly used today, few of which have been properly tested for safety. Single photon emission computed tomography scans (SPECT scans) and MRI spectrometry brain scans show that brain dysfunction and damage are present in sufferers of MCS (Hillert, Musabasic, Berglund, Ciumas, Savic 2007) (Haley, R., 2008).

A 2009 research study used SPECT scans to measure changes in the brain during chemical exposures in patients with MCS. The study found that there was a decrease in neural activity in the area of the brain responsible for odour processing during chemical exposure, and that limbic system sensitization can be involved in the pathogenesis of MCS (Orriols, Costa, Jacas, Castell, Sunyer, 2009). Another study from 2013 used positron emission tomography (PET) scans to measure changes in brain function in patients with MCS and found that during chemical exposure, MCS patients had increased activation of the anterior cingulate cortex. MCS patients also had significantly higher harm avoidance and anxiety in an acoustic startle test (Hillert, L., Jovanovic, H., Ahs, F., Savic, I., 2013).

CHRONIC FATIGUE SYNDROME (CFS)

CFS, also known as myalgic encephalomyelitis, post-viral fatigue syndrome, or chronic fatigue immune dysfunction syndrome, is characterized by relentless fatigue that does not improve with rest. A recent study of the occurrence of CFS in the United States estimates from .2% to above 2% or from 627,800 to above 6,278,000 cases. This same percentage estimates that from 70,000 to 700,000 Canadians are living with CFS (Wyller, V.B., 2007).

Symptoms of CFS include post-exertion malaise, unrefreshing sleep, widespread muscle and joint pain, sore throat, headaches of a type not previously experienced, cognitive difficulties, chronic, often severe, mental and physical exhaustion, and other characteristic symptoms in a previously healthy and active person. Persons with CFS may report additional symptoms including muscle weakness, increased sensitivity to light, sounds, and smells, orthostatic intolerance, digestive disturbances, depression, and cardiac and respiratory problems.

The symptoms of CFS can result in severely reduced participation in daily activities. Sufferers are primarily female (3:1). CFS is a limbic system condition triggered by neurological trauma which may involve viral, environmental, and/or psychological factors. The way in which the brain, mind, and body express this trauma is unique to each person. Many symptoms may overlap with those listed for MCS.

FIBROMYALGIA (FM)

Fibromyalgia is a medical disorder characterized by chronic widespread muscle and joint pain, inflammation, and allodynia (a heightened and painful response to pressure). Many complain of a host of other symptoms, including headaches, insomnia, irritable bowel syndrome, and chronic fatigue. Fibromyalgia is frequently present with conditions such as depression and anxiety, and with stress-related disorders such as PTSD.

In some cases, symptoms gradually accumulate over time with no single triggering event. Symptoms can be aggravated by noise, weather changes, and stress. The way in which the brain, mind, and body express this trauma is unique to each person.

ELECTRIC HYPERSENSITIVITY SYNDROME (EHS)

EHS is an environmental illness resulting in hypersensitivity to electromagnetic fields (EMFs). The symptoms of EHS include headache, fatigue, anxiety, sleep disturbances, skin symptoms like prickling, burning sensations, and rashes, pain and ache in muscles, abdominal pain, metallic taste and many other symptoms related to exposure to electromagnetic fields. EHS frequently occurs in patients who have MCS, and many symptoms may overlap.

Due to the growing presence of EMFs in the environment from modern electronics, those who suffer from severe EHS are often forced to live outside of buildings, or even away from society at large, to avoid triggers. Sufferers are often unable to use most modern technology including TV, computers, cell phones or wireless technology.

Given the breadth of health affects resulting from limbic system dysfunction, it is understandable that many traditional and alternative methods are generally limited in treating these conditions. While I recognize that toxins in our environment can be the cause of initial trauma to the limbic system, understanding how neuroplasticity is both at the root of suffering and the path to recovery is essential in treating limbic system-related conditions, and many mysterious and chronic illnesses.

CHAPTER 4

Why Traditional Therapeutic Techniques Don't Work

In a traditional psychotherapeutic model, a therapist works with an otherwise healthy patient to process a painful trauma, prompting the neural networks associated with this trauma to enter a heightened neuroplastic state. This state has the highest physical capacity for creating change, both positive and negative, by reorganizing neural circuits. When a patient goes back to an initial painful experience, however, the brain typically travels the same neural pathways that are associated with that memory. However, when the experience is addressed from a therapeutic perspective of understanding, compassion, self-love, and empowerment, a different emotional response and a different understanding of this experience can be generated.

In doing so, the associations to that memory are changed. This change in emotional charge also determines which neuropeptides will be released whenever this memory is recalled. Neuropeptides are chemical information messengers that allow all cells in the body to communicate with each other. This includes brain-to-brain messages, brain-to-body messages, body-to-body messages, and body-to-brain messages. This process of altering the emotional charge transforms the meaning and understanding of the trauma, thereby disengaging the threat and pain perception that was neurologically associated with it. At the physical level, a reorganization of neural circuits occurs, allowing the experience to be moved from its place as an on-going issue in the present, to the past, where it belongs.

However, this typical therapeutic model does not work in the patient suffering from a limbic system condition for a number of reasons. In a limbic system condition, the threat mechanism is stuck in the 'on' position, and all experiences are unconsciously perceived through the lens of threat. When a past traumatic event is brought into consciousness, the brain does not have the ability to address the experience appropriately. Due to the high levels of stress hormones associated with a limbic system condition, the patient is already in a state of trauma. Engaging in memories or strategies that focus on recounting the past trauma is counterproductive, as the brain does not have the ability to shift the trauma into the past. For example, this is commonly seen in cases of PTSD. In order for neural circuits to change, the limbic system needs to move out of its chronic alarm state and into a more relaxed state where growth and repair are possible. Typical therapeutic processes that involve uncovering emotions such as pain, fear, anger, resentment, or hopelessness are not recommended for the patient suffering from limbic system dysfunction. Due to their condition, the patient is not capable of healthy processing of a traumatic event. Rather, the treatment is likely to reinforce the patient's trauma.

Every time we consciously engage the patient in memories or experiences associated with the trauma, we are actually re-engaging the neurological pathways that are involved with the threat mechanism and reinforcing the threat. Even if a new intellectual understanding of the experience is temporarily attained, the brain is unable to process this new perception and will ultimately revert to the dysfunctional 'threat' patterns that are characteristic of limbic system conditions. Negative thoughts and emotions, as well as the repetitive nature of these feelings, can be symptomatic of limbic system dysfunction, and entertaining these emotions can actually reinforce the pathological neural pathways.

A comprehensive understanding of limbic system dysfunction is essential for productive treatment. The very real physical suffering and breakdown of multiple systems associated with this set of illnesses must be taken into account. Without this, traditional situations where the expectations of the therapeutic process hang so heavily on the patient's willingness and ability to change may actually result in further trauma. This can lead to further feelings of misunderstanding, failure, and hopelessness.

TOXIC OVERLOAD

It is thought that in illnesses like chronic fatigue syndrome, fibromyalgia, multiple chemical sensitivity, and post-traumatic stress disorder, there is an overproduction of nitric oxide (NO) and its product peroxynitrite (ONOO) known as the NO/ONOO cycle (Pall, M., 2007). This potent oxidant is produced in response to temporary and long-term stressors such as bacterial, fungal and viral infections, pesticides, organic solvents, or severe psychological stress that can initiate chronic illness.

Brain imaging studies have shown that "high concentrations of nitric oxide (NO) are found in brain regions involved in the modulation of anxiety and defensive behavior (Vincent and Kimura 1992) and exposure to stressful stimuli has been found to induce the activation of NO-producing neurons in the amygdala, hypothalamus, peri-aquaductal grey, and pedunculopontine tegmental nucleus (Krukoff and Khalili, 1997) (Oosthuizen, F., Wegener, G.,Harvey, B. H., 2005).

While I agree with this research on the affects of nitric oxide and peroxynitrite on brain function and physiology, I believe this chronic illness cycle can be interrupted through top-down regulation by rewiring limbic system structure and function. Given that the brain is constantly producing specific combinations of chemicals for every given event and reaction, and that rewiring the limbic system causes a change in that chemical production, a logical conclusion is that rewiring the limbic system would also act on the production of NO and ONOO and break the cycle. As discussed below, two approaches to controlling NO and ONOO are to use nutritional supplements and to engage in detoxification processes to cleanse the body of noxious substances. Although the addition of nutritional supplements may affect the NO/ONOO cycle, supplementation does not address the underlying issue of the overactive threat mechanism or the ongoing overproduction of NO. Furthermore, given the volatile state of the limbic system when injured and malfunctioning, it is important to approach the treatment of any underlying conditions such as toxic overload, viruses, fungi, or bacteria with caution, so as not to further activate the threat mechanism already in play. While detoxification treatments may be beneficial in some cases of ill-health, it is important to acknowledge that limbic system dysfunction can affect detoxification processes.

VAGUS NERVE

The vagus nerve originates in the brain and is the 10th cranial nerve. It runs from the hypothalamus through the chest and diaphragm to your intestines and has many different branches that relay signals between the brain and various body systems to regulate heart rate, speech, sweating, blood pressure, glucose production, and certain aspects of breathing. The vagus nerve is crucial for healthy digestion, and it is what creates our 'visceral' feelings about our experiences. It helps the body respond to stress and is central to homeostasis and to one's overall well-being. It plays a role in health restoration, cell regeneration, body detoxification, digestion and self-protection. It is thought that healthy innervation of the vagus nerve is linked with improved neurogenesis (creation of new brain or neuronal cells), and increased production of the neurotransmitter responsible for neurogenesis, namely brain-derived neurotrophic factor.

Trauma to the limbic system can cause chronic inflammation in the central nervous system, thereby keeping the brain and body stuck in a pattern of disease, or a 'limbic system trauma loop.' The chemical combination produced in the brain associated with a limbic system disorder and the resulting trauma loop actually prevents the vagus nerve from functioning properly. It is important to note that excessive activation of the vagus nerve during emotional stress, which is an overcompensation response associated with the stress response, can also cause fainting because of a sudden drop in blood pressure and heart rate.

Research has found that healthy innervation of the vagus nerve activates the neurotransmitter acetylcholine, which dampens the inflammatory process (Sloan et al. 2007) (Pavlov, T., 2005). Acetylcholine is also beneficial for creating a state of relaxation, which is crucial for learning and memory. The deactivation of threat mechanisms is required for learning or memory formation, which is incredibly difficult under extreme stress. Acetylcholine helps to 'reset' the internal alarm system after being triggered by a perceived threat. The vagus nerve relays to the rest of the body that it is safe to return to its normal resting/regenerative state. Healthy vagus nerve innervation also provides stability to the immune system. With a limbic system impairment, the function of the vagus nerve is negatively affected as the brain is in a constant state of threat. However, with limbic system reorganization, the vagus nerve can return to normal function.

The vagus nerve also affects liver function and detoxification processes. Recent research has implicated the vagus nerve in the cytochrome P450 pathway, the predominant enzyme system in phase 1 detoxification in the liver (Ashirmetov AKh, Krakovskiï, 1990). It is not uncommon for patients with limbic system disorders to be unable to process prescription drugs or nutritional supplements due to poor functioning of their detoxification and filtering systems. Often patients will become sensitive to the substances, making it impossible for them to take them.

The inability to clear toxins may lead to brain disorders, autoimmunity, chronic inflammatory conditions, chronic pain, and adrenal dysfunction as well as many other potential imbalances. Interestingly, toxic overload can be both the cause of and a symptom of limbic system dysfunction, proving that the relationship between the brain and detoxification processes is a two-way street. It would follow then that limbic system reorganization would encourage healthy detoxification processes.

In her book, *The Last Best Cure*, Donna Jackson Nakazawa notes that "although many medicines can temporarily dampen the sympathetic system, including anti-anxiety drugs such as valium and some antidepressants, there are no medications we can take to boost the parasympathetic nervous system." (Jackson Nakazawa, 2013). Patrica L. Gerbarg, MD and Richard Brown, MD, have found that stimulating the vagus nerve and parasympathetic nervous system through yoga breathwork helps to build stress resilience (Brown, R. P., Gerbang, P. L., 2012). The Dynamic Neural Retraining System™ effectively stimulates the parasympathetic nervous system in a similar way, allowing the brain and body to return to a normal resting state.

WHAT'S MISSING IN DETOXIFICATION, SUPPLEMENTATION AND AVOIDANCE?

Typical forms of treatment for limbic system impairments include detoxification of heavy metals, nutritional supplements, and avoidance. While detoxification methods may decrease the toxic load in the body, this does not address the underlying limbic system dysfunction. In fact, at times, detoxification can be too aggressive for the patient suffering from limbic system conditions and can cause an increase in symptoms. This is a challenge for a healthy system, let alone one that is in 'survival mode' where detoxification processes are already compromised. Equally, nutritional supplements may support various systems of the body, but they ultimately do not alter limbic system function. Often, as the list of sensitivities grows, sufferers will become hypersensitive to remedies or nutritional supplements, making them impossible to take. As noted earlier, this is also true for many prescribed pharmaceutical medications.

In addition, it is important to be careful with treatments that may cause additional stress on the central nervous system. Directly attacking latent infections or modulating the immune system can cause excessive stimulation of the sympathetic nervous system, in turn adding to limbic system stimulation. Many 'energizing' supplements or detoxification treatments can contribute to nervous system hypersensitivity as well. Additionally, even though co-infections may have been aggressively treated, and the pathogens no longer remain in the body, the brain can still be stuck in a 'fight-or-flight' state which expresses itself as lingering symptoms of illness. While these treatments are often supportive and necessary, patients will often not fully recover until the abnormal stress response is also addressed.

Although some may try a great many alternative practices,

the most common recommendation for patients suffering from limbic system dysfunction is to avoid that which triggers the symptoms. Up until now, avoidance has been the most logical behaviour in response to symptoms. However, this approach needs to be reexamined in a new light with the understanding of the plastic properties of the brain and how it changes in response to trauma. This understanding of how environmental triggers can alter brain structure and function is an essential part of the recovery process. The first set of truths: We know that environmental exposures to common chemicals, pesticides, viruses, bacteria, and electromagnetic fields can be dangerous to our health. We know that these exposures are often the cause of limbic system trauma. We also know that toxic overload is known to be associated with many illnesses like chemical sensitivities, chronic fatigue syndrome, and fibromyalgia. What we see in these conditions are the consequences of our global industrialization as reflected in human illness. The environmental impact that we can see throughout the planet is also severely affecting humans who are part of that environment. All of this is common knowledge, and therefore proactive environmental awareness is an essential part of illness prevention and overall health.

The other truth is that limbic system trauma has a profound affect on the central nervous system and on brain function, and as a result, it can alter our sensory perception. While complete avoidance of triggers may prevent symptoms temporarily, in the long run, avoidance can actually reinforce the pathological neural pathways that are in play with these conditions. In the "neurons that fire together – wire together" model, every time a specific encounter is avoided out of fear, the threat response to that stimulus is heightened. While we need to keep personal chemical and electromagnetic exposure and their environmental impact in mind, total avoidance will not change the dysfunctional mechanism.

An excellent example of perpetuating neural dysfunction through fear and avoidance behaviours is Leo DiCaprio's method acting technique for his role as Howard Hughes in the movie *Aviator*. Under the tutelage of American psychiatrist, Dr. Jeffrey Schwartz M.D., DiCaprio studied the nuances of obsessive compulsive disorder (OCD) so well that he actually developed a mild case of OCD:

> *DiCaprio left* The Aviator *with an Oscar-nominated performance and perhaps a mild case of the disease. It reportedly took him about a year to get back to normal. And today, his willful descent into the illness and subsequent recovery represents one of the most dramatic public examples in our popular culture of neuroplasticity — the ability of the brain to change in shape, function, configuration or size (Volk, 2013).*

With limbic system impairment, we must relearn how to inhibit the trauma feedback loop and stress response. In other words, the internal threat and survival mechanisms need to be reset or normalized. Through cognitive reappraisal and relabeling of both the symptoms and the stimuli, we can begin the process of regulating limbic system function and stop the downstream effects of a chronic stress response. Understanding this key step is pivotal in the recovery process. This goes against the typical grain, especially when we have been taught by our medical system that we should listen to every pain that our body is sending. After all, isn't pain the body's way of saying that something is wrong? Perhaps it is. Or perhaps pain is sometimes part of a limbic system impairment that is holding the brain hostage in a pain and trauma cycle.

Studies involving cognitive reappraisal point to how our

thoughts and emotions activate the brain centers for higher learning that can dampen the overactivated fear centres of the brain and help to stop the chronic stress response that keeps the brain and body in a state of 'dis-ease' (Modinos, G., Ormel, J., Aleman, A., 2010). Another more recent study looked at how cognitive restructuring (a technique in cognitive behavioural therapy) demonstrated that cognitive reinterpretation of a stimulus can change the emotional response specifically with fear conditioning (Shurick, A. A., Hamilton, J. R., Harris, L. T., Roy, A. K., Gross, J. J., Phelps, E. A., 2012).

The ability to step into the role of the curious observer, or what Dr. Jeffrey Schwartz calls "the impartial spectator," (Schwartz, J. 1997) and to distance oneself emotionally from reactive states is mandatory if we seek to rewire limbic system function. This requires that we change our focus from the outer environment to focusing on how to strengthen alternative neural circuitry.

A final note: this book is not a substitute for attending a DNRS program. Theoretical knowledge in itself is not enough to create the desired changes. The process of changing neural circuits in the limbic system requires the correct implementation and repetition of this information in a specific format. Just as a physiotherapist will prescribe a specific set of exercises to rehabilitate an injured muscle, the DNRS program is designed to rehabilitate the limbic system. It is an experiential process that takes dedication, understanding, discipline, commitment, and focus.

CHAPTER 5

Developing the Dynamic Neural Retraining System

Like many others, I had been to an endless list of medical professionals, both allopathic (conventional) and alternative, and had even gone to spiritual healers looking for answers and healing. I had tried 'everything,' and just like others, I was often left feeling defeated and skeptical of anyone who claimed that they could help. Time and time again, my hopes had been dashed and trying new treatments had largely proven to be costly – financially, emotionally, and physically. I had tried all the 'new age' positive thinking approaches and felt completely invalidated in my suffering. Any counseling efforts left me with the feeling of hopelessness or that the illness was in my head. The spiritual part of me wondered if I should just accept the condition as permanent and stop looking for answers.

I am so glad that I didn't stop looking. Far from being fictitious, I had suffered from a mild traumatic brain injury, and my brain was actually stuck in a trauma loop that was affecting all systems of my body. All of the positive thinking in the world was not enough to change the illness. What did help was my gradual understanding of limbic system dysfunction and applying the tools that I learned to retrain my limbic system.

Over the course of illness, I researched tirelessly, trying to find an explanation for my illness. I discovered a part of myself that I did not know existed before. Being in survival can make one extremely creative. I became an incessant and obsessed researcher. Certainly, if I was still healthy, I would not have been interested in brain science to this degree, but lo and behold, it was consuming all my waking moments. I was introduced to many aspects of neuroplasticity and was convinced that neuroplasticity held the answers I was looking for.

WHAT IS NEUROPLASTICITY?

According to Wikipedia, "Neuroplasticity, also known as brain plasticity, is an umbrella term that encompasses both synaptic plasticity and non-synaptic plasticity — it refers to changes in neural pathways and synapses which are due to changes in behavior, environment and neural processes, as well as changes resulting from bodily injury. Neuroplasticity has replaced the formerly held position that the brain is a physiologically static organ, and explores how – and in which ways – the brain changes throughout life."

The idea of brain function being involved in both the cause and possible resolution of my illness made sense to me and felt 'right' on a visceral level. A very instrumental book that was part of my healing is *The Brain That Changes Itself* (2007) by Dr. Norman Doidge. In this book, Doidge writes about a number of leaders in the field of neuroplasticity.

In the first chapter, Doidge speaks to the contributions of Dr. Paul Bach-y-Rita, an American neuroscientist who was a pioneer in the field of neuroplasticity and who introduced sensory substitution as a tool to treat patients suffering from neurological disorders. When describing one of Bach-y-Rita's patients, who had a damaged vestibular system (sense of balance), Doidge writes, "Cheryl Schiltz feels like she is perpetually falling" (Doidge, N., 2007, Pg. 1).

Through use of a sensory substitution device, Cheryl was able to relearn balance again through recruiting other parts of her brain. This breakthrough was remarkable and also an example of how the brain will find a way to compensate for lost function when given the right stimulus. With assistance from the device, Cheryl's brain created new neural pathways to restore balance. Over time, she no longer needed the device because her brain had naturally re-wired itself.

Although my own health problem was not about balance, I could relate to this story in some ways. Instead of feeling like I could never find my balance, I felt that my entire life was consumed with a feeling of impending threat and a need for safety. This was my twenty-four-hours-a-day, seven-days-a-week job. Just as Cheryl Schiltz constantly felt like she was falling, a person with a limbic system disorder feels like they are constantly in a state of survival. Further along in the same chapter, Doidge states, "We have senses we don't know we have until we lose them" (Doidge, N., 2007, Pg. 3). Similarly, I realized that, with limbic system disorders, we have senses we don't know we have until they are altered or heightened.

In *The Brain That Changes Itself*, Dr. Norman Doidge recounts his discussion with Dr. Bach-y-Rita about the brain's ability to change and adapt:

> *A brain system is made of many neuronal pathways, or neurons that are connected to one another and working together. If certain key pathways are blocked, then the brain uses older pathways to go around them. "I look at it this way," says Bach-y-Rita. "If you are driving from here to Milwaukee, and the main bridge goes out, first you are paralyzed. Then you take old secondary roads through the farmland. Then, as you use these roads more, you find shorter*

paths to use to get where you want to go, and you start to
get there faster." These "secondary" neural pathways are
"unmasked," or exposed and with use strengthened. This
"unmasking" is generally thought to be one of the main
ways the plastic brain reorganizes itself (Doidge, 2007, Pg. 9).

Upon further research and understanding of limbic system function, I surmised that disorganization of neural circuits in the limbic system were most likely at the root of the symptoms I was experiencing. The idea that the limbic system could be involved in distorted sensory perception was brought home by Jill Bolte Taylor's book, *My Stroke of Insight*, where she writes:

We are all unique in how much stimulation is required
before we can smell or taste something. Each of these sen-
sory systems is also made up of a complex cascade of cells,
and damage to any portion of the system may result in an
abnormal ability to perceive (Bolte Taylor, 2008, Pg. 21).

One of the most important developments in neuroscience over the past few decades is the development of neuroimaging techniques such as high-resolution magnetic resonance imaging (MRI), functional magnetic resonance imaging (fMRI), positron emission tomography (PET), and single photon emission tomography (SPECT). These technologies have promoted the identification of structural and functional characteristics underlying multiple chronic conditions. It is this body of research, combined with my own experience and my research, that led me to the conclusion that I had most likely suffered from a toxic brain injury that affected the limbic system in my brain. I postulated that my brain was stuck in a survival/fear loop and that this mechanism was likely at the root of all of my suffering. This made much more sense when I started to look at the research on fear mechanisms in the brain and how they are related to chronic stress and the development of disease.

From what I could gather, neural networks in my limbic system were altered as a result of trauma, and this disorganization or cross wiring of neural networks was playing havoc with my brain and body. My brain was unconsciously reacting to stimuli in my environment without my conscious awareness. During the initial trauma, my brain had created the association between chemicals and trauma, and subsequently, anything that was remotely similar to the initial injury triggered a severe toxic threat response. It had somehow wired any perception of chemicals with profound trauma, which triggered the 'get the heck out of here before you die' pathway. The more these mis-wired pathways fired, the stronger they became. The stronger they became, the worse my physical reaction became. The worse the reaction, the more the sensitivities spread. It wasn't long before I was enmeshed in this looping cycle with an ever expanding list of sensitivities and symptoms.

Also featured in *The Brain That Changes Itself* is the work of Donald Hebb, a Canadian psychologist responsible for the theory behind the concept of "neurons that fire together – wire together":

> *In 1949 Hebb proposed that learning linked neurons in new ways. He proposed that when two neurons fire at the same time repeatedly (or when one fires causing another to fire) chemical changes occur in both, so that the two tend to connect more strongly (Doidge, 2007, Pg. 63).*

This aspect of neuroplasticity is a property of the brain that is involved in all learning. It is also a key player in the type of brain dysfunction which is responsible for the tenacity of trauma-induced brain patterns. Of equal importance is the fact that neuroplasticity is the primary factor in limbic system rehabilitation and recovery.

When I got to the chapter in *The Brain That Changes Itself* about Dr. Jeffery Schwartz and his work with patients who had obsessive-compulsive disorder, it all started to make sense, and I had a big "aha!" moment. Dr. Schwartz made a considerable contribution to the field of neuroplasticity with the book *Brain Lock, Free Yourself from Obsessive-Compulsive Behavior, a Four Step Self-Treatment Method to Change Your Brain Chemistry*, written with Beverly Beyett. Dr. Schwartz discovered that the caudate, a structure in the brain involved in moving one thought to another, was not functioning properly in patients with obsessive-compulsive disorder. Dr. Schwartz referred to this as *brain lock*. With an OCD attack, patients were completely fixated on a feeling of dread and worry and became caught in behaviours that were driven by this 'locked' mechanism. Even though they didn't want to perform the behaviours, they felt that they could not stop themselves. Performing the behaviour would temporarily decrease their worry, but in the long run, it would actually make the condition worse. Dr. Schwartz surmised that if paying attention to the worry strengthened the pathological neural circuits at play and made the illness worse, then the opposite could also be true. If his patients could distract themselves from compulsive worrying by focusing on something pleasurable, then logically this should cause positive structural changes in the brain and weaken the neural circuits responsible for symptoms of OCD.

The more the patients continued to focus on a pleasurable feeling during an OCD attack, the more they created new neural circuits. For the patients, this was easier to understand when they were shown pictures of their brain during an OCD attack. They could look to the brain as the source of their discomfort and not their external environment. In understanding that their symptoms were initiated in the brain, and through constant, conscious attention, the patients strengthened the new neural circuits that eventually overrode the older pathological circuits at the heart of the illness. In so doing, they changed the structure and function of their brains. Eventually, the symptoms of illness decreased, and the patients learned how to control the illness, rather than being victims of it.

It was this new understanding of brain function and neuroplasticity that was ultimately a huge milestone in the development of the Dynamic Neural Retraining System™. When looking at my own situation in this new light, I considered the possibility that my symptoms were a result of limbic system dysfunction rather than a host of unrelated physical reactions. What if my brain was sending my body false messages? If the feelings associated with OCD were rooted in brain function, then was it possible that the numerous sensitivities, chronic pain, and inflammation that I was suffering from were also rooted in brain function? If OCD could be changed through focusing attention away from the worry and thereby altering brain function, then could I similarly override the feeling of threat? Maybe avoidance wasn't the only answer. Maybe I could actively take control of my brain and the symptoms. What if I could retrain my brain to function in a different way? Would this change the associated heightened sensory perception?

Another key concept brought up by Dr. Schwartz was the act of relabeling the symptoms. Recognizing the symptoms as a malfunction of the brain rather than as a characteristic of the stimulus was monumental. It shifted the focus from constantly trying to avoid exposures and triggers which were essentially uncontrollable and brought the focus toward something that was potentially controllable: I could choose how to focus my attention.

Similar to OCD, limbic system disorders tend to strengthen over time and can alter the structure and function of the brain. Also like OCD, a patient suffering from a limbic system disorder has mechanisms in the brain that keep it stuck in specific threat and protection patterns. The person with OCD gets stuck in a feeling of dread that something bad is going to happen and engages in repetitive behaviours in an attempt to stop the feeling, such as constantly washing their hands due to a feeling of contamination by germs. Although obsessive hand washing may relieve some anxiety in the short term, OCD sufferers are reinforcing the dysfunctional neural network. The more they acquiesce to their behaviour, the stronger the feeling of dread becomes, intensifying their feelings of helplessness. Comparing this information to my own situation actually made a lot of sense to me, and it explained why avoidance initially would make me feel safe and prevent symptoms of illness, but in the long run would make the condition much worse.

However, for the person who suffers from a limbic system disorder, the cause of symptoms is usually related to trauma. In MCS, there is likely a toxic chemical exposure or mould exposure that caused the initial brain trauma that causes the impaired threat mechanism to constantly fire.

Unlike OCD, where the patient is worried about potential harm that may seem irrational, with MCS the fear is quite rational. There is an undeniable truth that chemicals in our environment are dangerous to the brain and body. This is also true for electromagnetic fields, mould, bacteria, fungus and viruses. This knowledge is founded on scientific research and cannot be disputed. However, with limbic system dysfunction, what must be kept in mind is that sensory perception is distorted due to a threat mechanism in the brain that has gone awry. This causes the misinterpretation of minute quantities of stimuli as potentially life threatening.

Due to the perpetual sense of threat and survival, my amygdala was constantly overfiring. In a threat situation, the amygdala – the fear center of the brain – would normally be activated only when necessary. With a limbic system disorder, it is likely overactivated by the malfunctioning anterior cingulate cortex which keeps the brain focused on the perceived threat.

Living in a constant state of threat or survival activates the hypothalamus-pituitary-adrenal axis, resulting in excess production of stress hormones. This causes the body to activate protective mechanisms in every system in the body down to the cellular level. It moves the body from a state of growth and repair into a state of protection. The body becomes incapable of activities that are associated with rest and digestion, absorption, detoxification, and cell-to-cell communication. The brain continually takes cues from the body, sensing particular levels of hormones, which confirms a continued state of crisis, and the cycle becomes a negative feedback loop.

In the case of chemical sensitivities, this can result in an extremely heightened sense of smell that enables patients to detect minute amounts of potentially dangerous chemicals in the environment, even from great distances. Their heightened ability to smell enables them to detect the smallest of particles. The quality of smells can become acrid and bitter, leaving a foul taste in the mouth. Patients will often feel like they are literally being poisoned. Symptoms from exposure to chemicals in everyday fragrant products like perfume, cleaning agents, or chemicals that are off-gassing from carpets or new furniture can range from headaches and cognitive impairment to complete exhaustion and seizures. As this cycle continues, the sense of smell becomes more dominant, and the patient uses this sense as a warning signal. This can also occur with the sense of taste. Also of note is that the sense of smell is the only sense that is processed directly by the limbic system. For the patient with chemical sensitivities, the sense of smell would typically begin to take up more physical space in the brain, thereby changing the 'brain map' for the sense of smell and taste. Occasionally, it is also possible that patients can lose their sense of smell altogether.

Likewise, in the case of chronic fatigue syndrome, it may be a virus that triggers limbic system dysfunction. Although the virus may be latent, the brain becomes stuck in a protective pattern triggered by the virus. In post-traumatic stress disorder, the protective brain pattern is triggered by a crushing psychological trauma. The brain is simply unaware that the impending threat is no longer present. Whether the trigger is caused by toxic trauma, psychological stress, emotional trauma, viral, bacterial or fungal infection doesn't matter. The brain becomes stuck in a rogue threat mechanism that activates a chronic stress response that can affect both the brain and the body. The associated unconscious reactions and non-use of filtering mechanisms become re-enforced and strengthened over time.

TOXIC TRAUMA AND BRAIN MAPPING

It made sense to me that toxic trauma could alter brain mapping in a variety of ways. As I continued to investigate the work of neuroplasticity experts and continued to look at brain studies such as functional MRIs and SPECT scans, I found evidence of shared brain dysfunction in many related and overlapping conditions. This confirmed my hypothesis that limbic system dysfunction was the common denominator.

The idea that brain mapping could be altered with trauma was supported in *The Brain That Changes Itself* when Dr. Doidge describes the work of Dr. Michael Merzenich, an American neuroscientist who refers to brain patterns associated with dysfunction as "brain map-processing issues":

> *if [brain] maps could change, thought Merzenich, then there was reason to hope that people born with problems in brain map-processing areas—people with learning problems, psychological problems, strokes, or brain injuries-might be able to form new maps if he could help them form new neuronal connections, by getting their healthy neurons to fire together and wire together (Doidge, 2007 Pg. 63).*

With Merzenich's work, the idea that I could recruit other parts of my brain to substitute for the parts that were not functioning properly gave me hope for healing.

This idea of being able to consciously change the brain was also supported by the work of Dr. Eric Kandel, an American psychiatrist and researcher who did groundbreaking work in reflexive, protective responses in relation to learned fear. Kandel won a Nobel prize in 2000 for his work that demonstrated that neurons alter their structure and increase the number of synaptic connections between them as we learn. For me, his work brought forward the possibility that, as we purposely alter our thought processes, emotional states, and behaviours, we can redirect the brain to take alternate pathways or to engage in different neural networks.

Another voice that supported the idea that I could change my physical health by changing my limbic system's unconscious and distorted reactions was that of Dr. Bruce Lipton, author of

The Biology of Belief. Dr. Lipton was interested in working with the subconscious mind but also at a level above genetics, aptly termed, epigenetics.

> *The science of epigenetics, which literally means "control above genetics" profoundly changes our understanding of how life is controlled (Pray 2004; Silverman 2004). In the last decade, epigenetic research has established that DNA blueprints passed down through genes are not set in stone at birth. In other words, genes are not destiny! Environmental influences, including nutrition, stress, and emotions, can modify those genes without changing their basic blueprint. And those modifications, epigenticists have discovered, can be passed on to future generations as surely as DNA blueprints are passed on via the double helix (Reik and Walter 2001; Surani 2001). (Lipton, 2005, Pg. 37)*

This was another mind-blowing revelation for me. Looking at the work of these notable scholars, it became apparent to me that the expression of genes was related to the neurotransmitters in the brain, and therefore could be changed through our conscious awareness. It was possible to consciously wire my brain for healing!

CONSCIOUS AWARENESS WAS NOT ENOUGH

With avoidance, it seemed as though I could manage to prevent symptoms, but this was not a practical solution. The only way to avoid exposures was to isolate myself, which was not conducive to my psychological or emotional health. Despite my best efforts to avoid exposures, my condition continued to deteriorate, and the illness progressed.

If a rogue fear mechanism was keeping my brain and body stuck in this cycle of illness, I wondered what I could do beyond avoidance that might relieve the symptoms. With this in mind I started to investigate what internal thoughts, feelings, and behavioural patterns were related to this feeling of threat or protection. Later on I would classify these patterns as 'pathways of the past,' or POPs.

In limbic system-related conditions, the brain has learned a sort of "non-use" or a malfunctioning of filtering mechanisms due to disorganization or cross wiring of neural circuits. This can alter our psychological processes, our emotional states, our behaviours, the function of the systems of our bodies, and even sensory perception, both internal and external. With limbic system dysfunction, the brain stops filtering information as it normally would. It sends erroneous and distorted messages and can no longer be trusted as the conveyor of truth. The idea that pain is the body's way of sending a message that something is wrong can no longer be trusted.

The idea that my brain could be sending my body false messages was mind-blowing. After all, I was completely focused on my symptoms and acutely listening to the messages that my body was sending me in an attempt to prevent further illness. I thought that the symptoms were a great warning sign of potential danger and were my cue to get away from the triggers/stimuli. To entertain this outlandish idea that the brain was sending incorrect alert messages was completely counterintuitive. My entire focus had been about disease, symptoms, and an ever-expanding knowledge base about toxins in our environment – all of which completely validated the illness. After all, wasn't I just a canary in the coal mine, warning others of impending doom? I struggled to fit these pieces of the puzzle together. In the end, I realized that while it is true that we have far too many sources of toxic stress in our environment, and it is true that toxic trauma can be the cause of limbic system impairment, ultimately, the limbic-impaired brain is not an accurate reporter. We must always be mindful of this and be prepared to work around it.

As a core belief counselor, I was very familiar with the process of being a curious observer. In my practice, my primary function was to identify trauma and the thoughts, feelings, and behavioural patterns (i.e. the belief systems) that it initiated. I would teach my clients how to resolve trauma through interrupting habitual thoughts, feelings, and behaviours that reinforced limiting beliefs. When applying this skill set to my own situation, identifying distorted emotional, behavioural, and thought patterns that represented symptoms of limbic system disorganization became a large part of the process of recovery. I recognized that these patterns were all part of the same limbic system trauma cycle. Even though the trauma reactions were unconscious, I could bring my conscious attention to patterns that might be contributing to the cycle. Examining my emotional states was part of this inquiry.

In the beginning, I would allow myself to entertain whatever emotion was surfacing in an attempt to release the emotion and move forward. The ability to label, feel, and integrate feelings was a skill that I was very practiced at. This skill set had served me well in the past, so I started to adapt this to my new situation.

At the time, I was living on a broken-down houseboat, isolated from society and the world that I loved. I did not have heat or running water and lived a very basic life. I was in a state of survival, my body was constantly reacting to both chemical and electromagnetic exposures, and I was in chronic pain much of the time. Understandably, I was feeling very depressed, helpless, and hopeless. My primary thought was "how will I survive?"

Later on I realized that simply being consciously aware of patterns that were associated with a limbic system trauma loop was not enough to change the neural patterns at play. However, it took me some time to get to this realization.

In order to stop the threat mechanism from firing, I needed to completely change a number of things. I needed to change my perspective about the stimuli, to alter my thought processes, to direct my emotional state on a moment-to-moment basis, and to change the self-protective behaviours that I had grown accustomed to. Previously, I had believed that the protective avoidance behaviours that I had cultivated were the only thing preventing me from further illness. Changing this attitude had seemed entirely counterintuitive. Dr. Joe Dispenza, author of *Breaking The Habit of Being Yourself*, discusses this reaction:

> *When our stress response is triggered we focus on three things and they are of highest importance. The body (it must be taken care of), the environment (where can I go to escape this threat) and time (how much of it do I have to use in order to evade this threat?). The stress response and the hormones that it triggers, force us to focus on (and stress about) the body, environment, and time. As a result, we begin to define our "self" within the confines of the physical realm; we become less spiritual, less conscious, less aware, and less mindful. ...Our identities become wrapped up in our bodies. (Dispenza, J., 2012, Pg. 100-101)*

In retrospect, I can see how much of my time (okay, *all* of my time) was spent thinking about symptoms (my body), what to avoid (the environment), and how quickly I could escape the danger (time). I was caught in a limbic system trauma loop. For support during this dark time, I would call my partner James and lament about the negative aspects of my day. At the time, it felt like support and important validation, which was invaluable. What I learned later on was that recounting all of the problems that I was facing and focusing on what I perceived to be a constant threat were reinforcing the cross wired neural patterns associated with trauma, thereby strengthening the limbic system disorder.

As a trained counselor, I thought it would be productive to process the emotions that were coming up. Feelings of sadness, abandonment, loss, grief, anger, fear, and worry were cycling in my mind. I would often find myself thinking about past trauma for no apparent reason. Additionally, when I thought of my isolating situation and the hopelessness that I felt with being ill, I thought that perhaps this was just a rerun of old childhood wounds and associated feelings. I mistakenly thought that investigating these feelings would help me move forward. However, over time I realized that entertaining the feelings made my symptoms much worse. Similar to Dr. Jeffery Schwartz's earlier observations about entertaining OCD thought patterns, my entertaining feelings associated with limbic system trauma was inevitably counterproductive, even though these feelings were inarguably valid given the reality of the situation. My brain was stuck in a perpetual feeling of threat, and I could not reason my way out of it. Even when I thought that I had come to a place of integrating the feeling and was able to take a different perspective, the same thoughts and feelings would appear ten minutes later. I felt like a gerbil on a wheel. After many boxes of Kleenex, many tearful journal entries, and negative thoughts like 'I'd rather be dead', it became evident to me that exploring these emotions was also not the answer.

My next step was simply to observe the patterns and not entertain them. I thought that I could simply detach myself from them and watch them float by. However, when your brain is stuck in a threat mechanism, it is challenging to distance yourself from thoughts and feelings or to ignore physical symptoms. It's a primitive, instinctual reaction that is not consciously driven. Being an impartial observer was not enough. At this point, I realized that my thoughts and emotions needed an intervention! Simply observing the pattern was not enough to change it – I had to find a way to get my brain out of the rogue threat mechanism. Just as Schwartz got his patients to actively interrupt the worry circuit, I had to find a way to interrupt the threat circuit. This required that I redirect my focus away from the trigger, the patterns, and any reactions. I had to keep my mind and emotions actively engaged in a different direction, away from fear.

The ability to step into the role of curious observer is a fundamental aspect in changing limbic system function. Dr. Bruce Lipton speaks to this skill set:

> *In its self-reflective capacity, the conscious mind can observe behaviors as they are being carried out. As a pre-programmed behavior is unfolding, the observing conscious mind can step in, stop the behavior, and create a new response. Thus the conscious mind offers us free will, meaning we are not just victims of our programming. To pull that off however, you have to be fully conscious lest the programming take over, a difficult task, as anyone who's tried will power can attest. Subconscious programming takes over the moment your conscious mind is not paying attention (Lipton, B H., 2005, Pg. 139).*

The ability to change my cognitive and emotional patterns, no matter what was going on, was a vital part of the recovery process. My first experience with this came very unexpectedly one dark, cold and rainy evening while living on the houseboat. The following is from an article that I wrote about that night.

"What I learned from my dog Bella"

My dog Bella is the cutest dog ever. I will admit that I am a bit biased; however she actually looks like a teddy bear, or if you can remember back to Star Wars, people often say she looks like an Ewok. She is an adorable four-legged soul with a very kind disposition – most of the time (unless you are knocking at the door in which case she morphs into a slobbering Doberman).

When Bella was a puppy, she had a favourite toy – Freddy the frog. She took Freddy the frog everywhere with her and would often plop Freddy down at my feet. No matter what, it was always a good time to play "throw the frog". Morning, noon or night, the commentary that ran through her head was "are you going to throw the frog now?"

Now let's flash back to 2007 when I was living on a houseboat sequestered by an illness to live in isolation and pain. Nightly I would phone my partner James for love and support during this difficult time.

Even though I had once considered myself to be a very positive person, the injury to my limbic system caused the survival and threat mechanisms in my brain to become hyperactive. As a result, it constantly felt like I was being poisoned by my environment or that I was constantly under attack. Some of my senses had also morphed into super-human powers to detect anything in my environ-

ment that could be a potential threat to my safety. My senses of smell and taste and my ability to detect electromagnetic fields had heightened in order to protect me from danger. As well, the associated maladapted stress response was causing breakdown of many of the systems of my body. My thoughts and emotional patterns were concerned with one thing only – my survival. Gone was the happy-go-lucky Annie that many had loved and cherished. As one can imagine, having a conversation with me would be enough to make anyone feel depressed.

One particularly cold and rainy evening, I was standing at the phone booth, making my nightly call to James to recount the daily war that I was engaged in. What he said to me on this particular night was both shocking and brilliant. It took me with such surprise that I asked him to repeat what he had said. As I stood in the rain, this trusted voice from the other end of the phone said, "Throw the Frog! Throw the Frog!"

In that moment, I realized what he was saying. Instantly I went from crying to laughing hysterically when I was reminded that I had the power to change the channel in my mind. And for that moment, I found relief in the laughter that had replaced the unrelenting survival pattern that my brain and body were stuck in.

As it turns out, learning how to shift out of survival patterns and learning to 'throw the frog' are just a part of the essential tools that we use to rewire limbic system function. However, when suffering from a limbic system impairment, this can seem like defying gravity itself and takes great understanding of brain function, immense dedication, persistence, and patience (Hopper, 2012).

I continued to experiment with trying to change my emotional state but realized that I had some resistance to going there. The following journal entry is from that time. At this point, I felt like I was fighting an emotional addiction with a unique combination of stress hormones and survival instincts.

From my journal 2007:

I can choose to feel something different. When have I felt the feeling that I desire? I can replicate this! I have to focus on thoughts and emotions that give me energy not take my energy. I am reminding myself to constantly surrender and look for the blessing. This almost seems contrived, but the other option is to continuously wallow in self-pity. Had enough of that – thanks anyway! During those times I feel helpless and hopeless. I sometimes forget that I have choice, especially when the darkness seems so real.

I have to look for evidence to support goodness. At times, I have found connection, compassion, love, understanding, comfort, ease, joy, laughter, support, peace, and fun.

So what is scary about going into a positive emotion? Because what if I discipline myself enough to go there and discover that it doesn't work? What if there is no warm and fuzzy feeling, but rather just a big void of vast emptiness? It's as if I can fool myself into believing there is something good, but if I go there I might find out that believing is really an illusion. Part of me would just rather sit and not do anything. But then I have to ask myself about the results that I am getting from sitting in this space. I am already experiencing what I fear the most, which is that feeling of emptiness, so really I have nothing to fear. When I engage in positive feelings, the glimmers of hope are ignited once again.

I WAS AFRAID TO HAVE HOPE

Looking back now, I realize that I was afraid to have hope. I didn't want to set myself up for disappointment again. I had tried so many different things in the past and nothing had helped. My mind also gravitated to spirituality and the thought of acceptance of my situation. I considered the idea that with a more spiritual perspective, I could find acceptance, gratitude, and happiness within my difficult circumstances. Maybe my life path was to warn other people of illness or promote environmental awareness?

When stuck in a state of illness for a long time, one can lose the ability to dream of being healthy. In fact, it seems dangerous to go there. The fear of disappointment and what feels like the inevitability of failure can severely inhibit one's engagement in the process of change.

If "neurons that fire together – wire together", then, I surmised, I should be able to create new neural connections by using highly charged positive emotional experiences. From here, I pushed myself to consciously remember times of joy, to recount positive memories, to focus on the good aspects of my life, and to cultivate a state of gratitude in a general way. At first, it felt really unnatural, foreign, and forced, especially in my chaotic situation. My brain did not want to go there. Although it felt counterintuitive to consciously change my thoughts and emotional state, I knew that staying where I was would only lead to more suffering. This was not the Pollyanna idea of 'positive thinking' that one might think. I recognized that the negative thought patterns were a symptom of limbic system trauma. My decision to stop entertaining them was not a form of denial but rather I was consciously directing and changing my thought patterns to act back on the brain in a very specific way. Equally,

I realized that my negative emotional states were also indicative of limbic system dysfunction. Consciously directing myself to a more positive emotional state was assisting in shifting the threat response. Periodically, I noticed that this new focus improved my symptoms overall.

However, the process of changing your emotional state is no easy task. Understanding why it may be difficult to get out of this pattern makes sense when we understand that the brain has an automatic negativity bias. If we do not feel safe and secure, the brain will naturally be on the lookout for potential danger in our environment. Our focus will be drawn to examine what is going wrong rather than notice what is going right. This is the brain's natural, self-protective state. As one can imagine, with a limbic system impairment, our perspective of the world becomes coloured with what is not going well. Even when we try to focus on what may be good in our lives, it feels strained and prescribed. Not only is our brain unaccustomed to looking for the good because it is in a limbic system trauma loop, the neural networks associated with joy are very weak. Furthermore, allowing oneself to be in a positive state makes one feel vulnerable to another disappointment.

This also makes sense when we understand that specific thoughts and feelings create very unique chemical formulas in the body. When they are repeated often enough, the brain and body perceive this chemical state as 'normal,' and it becomes our unconscious habit zone. The brain and body adapt to this state by creating more receptor sites on the cell walls that are designed to receive that unique chemical cocktail. We literally become addicted to a state of thinking and feeling (Pert, 1997).

Try as we may to think and feel differently, time and time again we find ourselves back in the rut. Just like any other addiction, this chemical cocktail will try to convince us to feed it. Any thought, feeling, or behaviour that does not match the unique chemical formula associated with the neural trauma pattern will feel unnatural and uncomfortable.

Because the brain registers this unnatural feeling as a threat to the body's status quo, we will unconsciously seek evidence to support staying in a rut or will find ways to justify our old thinking and feeling habits that feed the impairment. Dispenza speaks to this addiction when he writes, "trying to change your emotional pattern is like going through drug withdrawal" (Dispenza, J., 2012).

I recognized that my brain was addicted to survival-based hormones, and it would routinely pull my mind back to that habit zone with great tenacity. Overcoming habitual thought and emotion patterns associated with a limbic system trauma loop was a big challenge, yet doing so was essential to recovery. I had to learn to turn my focus away from symptoms of illness and toward the process of rewiring neural circuits. Often this meant that, in the middle of a reaction, I would have to take the stance of the curious observer, distance myself from the physical reactions and purposely change my emotional state. Although many of my symptoms were physical in nature and very painful, it was imperative for me to focus on consciously redirecting my brain.

UNDERSTANDING THE SCIENCE OF EMOTION

Understanding the science of emotion and reading *Molecules of Emotion* by Dr. Candace Pert helped me in this regard. Until Pert's work, emotions were thought to be location-specific and linked with emotional centers in the limbic system. While the limbic system is certainly involved in emotion, there are other emotional centres throughout the body. The chemical cocktail that is created from an emotion travels on neuropeptides and binds to emotion-specific receptor sites throughout the body. In effect, our emotions are constantly being processed by our bodies.

Ultimately, what I came to understand is that changing my emotional state was a major component in changing the wiring of my limbic system and thereby healing my body. The tools that I learned through Neural Linguistic Programming (NLP) helped me to further interrupt and block habitual neural patterns. When feelings of anxiety or fear would come up from symptoms of illness, or when I was around stimuli that would 'normally' trigger a reaction, I would consciously reframe the experience while anchoring myself in a positive emotional state. When I transformed my emotional state, I could actually feel the physical manifestation of the emotion throughout my brain and body. I could feel what I call the "warm and fuzzies" and a kind of tingling sensation through my head and body. When this happened, I knew that I was on the right track. Sometimes this would immediately shift the symptoms, and other times it would not. Either way, I figured I was going in the right direction. If the symptoms did not change, I avoided getting upset or angry as these feelings would simply feed the limbic system trauma loop. Rather, I simply trusted that, with repetition, I would strengthen alternative neural pathways.

MY PERSONAL LABORATORY

Please note that what I describe below was my personal process when developing the DNRS program and is not intended to be instructional in any way. I do not recommend trying this on your own. Without proper training and understanding of the Dynamic Neural Retraining System™, over-exposure to stimuli can be entirely counterproductive to recovery. Part of the practice is to systematically introduce challenges in a controlled and informed way. Please do not expose yourself to stimuli without first engaging in a DNRS program.

The next step for me was to test this theory, and the only way for me to do that was to consciously trigger myself in real life situations. Would it be possible to rewire my brain and body to react differently by consciously redirecting habitual patterns associated with a limbic system trauma loop while being triggered? I began to consciously put myself in situations that would 'normally' trigger symptoms. This took a great deal of courage and was not something that I entered into lightly. I cannot adequately relate how difficult this was or explain the leap of faith that this required, except to say that it was like defying gravity. The cost associated with triggers in the past was extreme, in terms of my immediate health; however, I was willing to try small exposures to see what happened. This took a lot of work, effort, and focus. It was decidedly uncomfortable, especially since I still had symptoms during this process. But over time, my brain relearned that the stimuli was not life-threatening. I learned how to filter information appropriately again, and my symptoms eventually started to fade. Occasionally I found that my sensory perception started to normalize. My sense of smell started to acclimatize to the stimulus rather than being repulsed by it. At first, I would notice a strong chemical smell, and eventually it would recede into the background. My sense of smell was adapting once again to the environment.

It was now time to start to incrementally train myself with bigger challenges. I wondered if I could adapt and apply the same training principles of constraint-induced movement therapy (CI therapy) as described in treating stroke patients by Dr. Doidge in *The Brain That Changes Itself*.

CI therapy was developed by Dr. Edward Taub, a behaviorist who became a brain researcher and worked with people who had suffered from strokes and had lost use of one of their arms. The focus of the therapy is to constrain the nonaffected arm with a heavy mitt, forcing the use of the affected limb. Through intensive therapy with a physical therapist, the patient is taught to use their seemingly paralyzed arm by doing simple, repetitive tasks with increasing difficulty. At first, the therapist assists the patient, while the patient focuses attention on small, repetitive, passive movements of their limb. Gradually, with extensive focus and repetition, the patient's brain learns to rewire itself to make up for lost function, and amazingly, the patient slowly begins to regain muscle function to perform the task unassisted. This incremental training process is known as *shaping*. CI therapy has also been used successfully in patients suffering from traumatic brain injury and cerebral palsy.

Was it possible for me to shape my own brain? I wondered if I could retrain my brain to filter incoming sensory stimulation in a normal and healthy way by introducing the 'offending' substance in small increments while staying focused on the fact that the reactions were coming from my brain, not the substance? What if I did this on a regular basis so that my brain became accustomed to using new neural pathways? This meant that my entire focus had to shift from avoidance to exposures, both planned and accidental, as opportunities to rewire my brain. This was not the same as 'pushing' myself through a challenging situation only to end up feeling more ill afterwards. This was very different. This approach was based on brain science and on reconditioning my brain.

With this new understanding, fear was removed from the equation, de-escalating the entire cycle. My brain was in the active process of rewiring itself. Within my limbic system, I surmised that changes were happening. The cingulate cortex stopped focusing so intensely on the perceived threat. This reduced the fear messages sent to the amygdala, which decreased the production of stress hormones in the pituitary and adrenal glands and calmed my entire system. Eventually, my sensory perception normalized, and my body resumed a state of homeostasis, returning to more healthy functions like growth and repair. My hippocampus had a chance to relearn the association to a particular stimulus, which helped to alleviate the anticipated fear. This prevented the cycle from reinitiating itself. My threat mechanism began to regulate itself. I had successfully changed the structure and function of my brain!

This was almost unbelievable as I had been to countless doctors with no lasting results and yet, I could direct my brain to work in a different way! It felt miraculous!

My state of health rapidly started to change when I understood that a faulty protective mechanism in my brain was triggering a chronic stress and inflammatory response in my body that also caused heightened sensory perception. I knew that applying all of these different aspects of neuroplasticity were fundamental for my own recovery. Simultaneously, I knew that my personal experience was essential to the development of the program. Even after integrating all of these elements, it took me a full six months of tireless dedication to recover. Having come through my own personal hell, I felt strongly about preventing others from having to experience the same kind of pain and invalidation that I did. I began to act on my personal promise to help others who were suffering. The culmination of all of these revolutionary ideas combined with my unique set of counseling and therapeutic skills led me to create what is now the Dynamic Neural Retraining System™. I'm grateful that the development of the program has also allowed me to pursue my life mission – to facilitate global healing while promoting a message of environmental awareness.

12 CRITICAL STEPS TO REWIRE THE LIMBIC SYSTEM

1. Develop awareness of the expression of limbic system dysfunction in physical, psychological, emotional, and behavioural patterns

2. Recognize and re-label symptoms as limbic system dysfunction

3. Interrupt patterns associated with limbic dysfunction

4. Decrease fear association to stimuli

5. Re-attribute symptoms to overactivated threat mechanism gone awry

6. Choose a new strategy for responding to stimuli

7. Cultivate a positive emotional state to dampen stress response

8. Cultivate a positive psychological state to retrain thought patterns associated with catastrophic thinking

9. Incrementally train yourself to strengthen new brain pathways and to systematically desensitize your response to the triggering stimuli

10. Change habits associated with extreme harm avoidance behaviour

11. Recognize improvements and celebrate them!

12. Repeat the new strategy daily for a minimum of an hour per day for 6 months

CHAPTER 6

Why the Dynamic Neural Retraining System™ Works

HOW STRESS AND TOXIC TRAUMA AFFECT THE BRAIN AND BODY

Stress can wreak havoc on the mind and body and is a big contributing factor to disease. We hear this often enough, but we rarely think of stress in any other form than psychological. Even more rarely do we think that our reaction to stress has a direct impact on our health and well being. Stress, in all of its forms, can be toxic to the brain at the physical, emotional, and psychological levels and can cause brain trauma. Stress also affects the body's ability to regulate inflammation (Cohen, S., Janicki-Deverts D., Doyle, W.J., Miller, G.E., Frank, E., Rabin, B.S., Turner, R., 2012).

Systemic inflammation is implicated in many chronic diseases and, not surprisingly, is also involved in limbic system conditions. While an acute trauma may cause the initial inflammation, it is the maladapted stress response involved with limbic system dysfunction that keeps the brain and body in a state of chronic inflammation. Psychological, emotional, and physical responses to stress are equally as important and can cause the brain to release a specific chemical cocktail that causes a chain of reactions in the body.

During a perceived threat situation, the brain sends a stress alert signal to the rest of the body. The adrenal glands, located on top of the kidneys, release adrenalin, also known as epinephrine. This increases heart rate, breathing, and blood pressure. It moves blood away from vital organs and into the extremities to prepare for 'fight-or-flight'. Senses become keener in a protective response in order to help assess the environment for impending threat. If the threat persists for more than a couple of minutes, the adrenals release cortisol. Cortisol remains in the body a lot longer than adrenalin and can damage brain cells, especially in the hippocampus, the area for memory and learning (Shin, L. M., Rauch, S. L., Pitman, R. K., 2006).

During this period of high stress, the body releases neurochemicals that increase sensory perception (sight, sound, smell, taste, touch) to protect oneself and to keep track of both real and perceived threat. After the threat has passed, the body stops producing neurochemicals that are associated with survival and returns to a natural resting state, and sensory perception returns to normal again.

In a healthy stress response, the hippocampus detects that the threat is no longer present and sends messages to the hypothalamus to stop releasing stress hormones and to start releasing calming hormones in order to bring the brain and body back into a state of balance, or homeostasis. However, this is not the case in conditions where there is limbic system dysfunction. The hippocampus no longer has a context for safety and sends inappropriate alarm messages to the hypothalamus to release more stress hormones. This becomes a negative feedback loop.

Stress can also increase the permeability of the blood-brain barrier, the complex system of blood vessels that protects the brain from toxins circulating in the blood stream. An example of this occurred during the Gulf War when Israeli soldiers were given a drug to protect themselves from chemical and biological warfare. Normally the drug should not have crossed the blood brain barrier; however, stress had somehow increased the permeability of the blood brain barrier resulting in symptoms associated with the drug itself, including nausea, headaches, and dizziness (Friedman, A. Kaufer, D., Shemer J., Hendler, I., Soreq, H., Tur-Kaspa I., 1996). Thus, it makes sense that the blood-brain barrier may be weakened in patients with limbic system dysfunction, leaving the brain more vulnerable to toxins.

Toxic trauma can also cause disruption in neuro-immune signaling, that is, in the connections between the brain and the immune system. When in a chronic stress response, the brain's immune cells, microglia, overreact. Microglia are basically white blood cells in the brain that represent the body's first line of immune defense, and their overreaction triggers the excessive secretion of cytokines that can cause pain and neural degeneration, increase inflammation, and alter gene expression (Watkins, L.R., Maier, S.F., 1999).

However, it is possible to influence the brain and body in a more positive direction. Dr. Steve Cole collaborated in a small, randomized, and controlled trial involving 40 adults. This research suggests that meditation can shift gene-expression away from pro-inflammatory genes and towards anti-viral genes (Creswell J.D., Irwin M.R., Burklund L.J., Lieberman M.D., Arevalo J.M., Ma, J., Breen E.C., & Cole S.W., 2012). This research furthers the idea that genes do not necessarily determine health. The expression of genes is influenced, in this instance quite positively, by mindfulness meditation. This opens the door for further research into what other influences may have similar affects.

Another study led by psycho-oncologist Michael Antoni at the University of Miami, Florida, involved 200 women with early-stage breast cancer. In those who completed a ten week stress management program, genes associated with inflammation and metastasis were down-regulated compared with those of women in the control group who simply attended a one day educational seminar. Additionally, genes involved in the type I interferon response which fights tumors as well as viruses were up-regulated in the women who took the stress management course (Antoni M.H., Lutgendorf SK, Blomberg B, Carver CS, Lechner S, Diaz A, Stagl J, Arevalo JM, Cole SW., 2012).

In additional to these stress management techniques, the ability to identify distorted reactions and to change our emotional state is pivotal in creating more positive neural networks. Although the limbic system is often considered to be the 'emotional brain,' there are a number of different places in the body that influence emotion and communicate with the brain. There are a number of positive feedback mechanisms active in the brain and body that favourably affect multiple systems in multiple ways. For example, oxytocin, a hormone produced primarily in the hypothalamus and secreted by the posterior pituitary gland, is associated with positive emotions involved with bonding and childbirth. Studies have shown that oxytocin down-regulates the hypothalamus-pituitary-adrenal axis involved in the chronic stress response. Evidence also suggests that oxytocin has a regulatory role during the immune and inflammatory responses (Clodi, M, Vila, G, Geyeregger, R., Riedl, M, Stulnig, T. M, Struck, J., Luger, T.A., Luger, A., 2008).

However, oxytocin is not only a hormone, it is also a neurotransmitter that directly modulates the release of cytokines (the chemical messengers that trigger inflammation). Oxytocin is produced in a number of areas in the body, not just in the brain. In fact, research has shown that many neurotransmitters involved in regulating the stress response are located in the nerve cell networks in the intestinal tract called the enteric nervous system. This area is so important in the regulation of various body functions that it has been dubbed 'the second brain.' Dr. Michael Gershon, chairman of the department of anatomy and cell biology at Columbia University and author of the book, *The Second Brain*, says that the brain in the head shares a unique connection with the brain in the gut. Gershon explains that 'the second brain' is equipped with neurotransmitters and the ability to control behaviour. Gershon found that oxytocin cools down gastrointestinal inflammation, which can be involved in conditions such as food disorders, autoimmune disorders, and systemic infections (Gershon, M.D.,Welch, M.G., Anwar, M., Chang, C.Y., Gross, K.J. Ruggiero, D.A, 2010). Thus, oxytocin has important beneficial effects on our health and our emotional well-being.

Oxytocin increases feelings of trust and bonding and decreases feelings of fear. Further, it can enhance your memory of bonding. There are natural ways to release oxytocin and the more you do it, the easier it becomes. The two most noted ways to release oxytocin are by engaging in sexual activity and in breast feeding. However, some more practical ways to increase blood levels of oxytocin are to create a sense of bonding by spending time with people, especially friends and loved ones, including pets, and by expressing your love and gratitude. Other methods are to relive positive memories, soak in a hot bath, give several hugs a day, and engage in social activities that bring you a sense of joy. Although there are many ways to release oxytocin, this alone is not enough to remap the limbic system and dampen a chronic stress response that has gone awry. However this will assist you in creating a fertile ground for neuroplastic changes to take hold in the brain.

Moving into a positive emotional state activates the communication between the heart and the brain and can influence function of higher brain centres involved in perception, cognition, and emotional processing. In the past, communication between these two organs has been thought of as one way – brain to heart. Research now suggests this is a two way dialogue and that the heart actually influences the brain in significant ways. Research suggests that initiating positive emotional states causes the heart and the brain to become synchronized, and this process can alter information processing in the brain in a positive way (McCraty, R. Atkinson, M., 1999).

Considerable research on this was completed by Dr. J. Andrew Armour, M.D. PhD, a neurologist at Centre of Research at Hôpital du Sacré-Coeur at the Université de Montréal, Canada. Armour discovered a large number of neurons in the heart, called sensory neurites, that communicate with the brain. He refers to these as "the little brain in the heart" (Armour, J.A., 2007). He notes that electromagnetic fields generated by the heart during a positive emotional state are much greater in intensity than the electromagnetic fields generated by the brain.

When we actively focus our attention away from perceived threat, we are activating the prefrontal cortex. This process does not occur with thought alone. When we consciously engage in positive emotional states such as joy, gratitude, a sense of awe, or love, the brain releases serotonin and other life-enhancing hormones and neurotransmitters that change the brain's internal chemical state. This creates a fertile environment for the brain to engage in developing alternate circuitry. As we learn to do this consciously, we weaken the pathological neural patterns associated with fear and pain that are overactivated in limbic system impairment.

Far from being merely 'positive thinking,' the process of rewiring limbic system function is a multifaceted process that takes great understanding and patience, and it also demands an understanding of how our everyday environment and other stressors contribute to disease. Over time, this new focus can change the deep wiring of the limbic system and normalize the signals that are being sent from the brain to the immune system. This affects both inflammation and the expression of genes that promote disease. According to epigenetics, the expression of genes are affected by neurotransmitters in our brain. If we have the ability to consciously change the internal environment of our brain and alter the hormones that we produce, it makes sense that in doing so, as Dr. Lipton surmises, we may be able to change the expression of genes (Lipton, 2005).

What this ultimately means is that what you think and how you feel matters. Understanding how a limbic system impairment alters threat perception and how this in turn affects overall health is a very big step in rewiring limbic system function. Given the right tools, it is possible to rewire the limbic system and thereby stop the chronic inflammatory response, allowing the brain and body to move from a state of 'fight-or-flight' into a state of rest, relaxation, and regeneration, where growth and healing can take place.

HOW AN OVERACTIVATED THREAT MECHANISM CAN LEAD TO ILLNESS

Stress reactions are often unconscious. An internal threat response can occur without the patient's conscious awareness of the stimulus that evoked it. Dr. Barry Gilbert comments on this unconscious processing of our environment in the article, "The Neurobiology of Anxiety." Gilbert examined the reaction within parts of the amygdala of people with high trait anxiety (people who are characteristically easily stressed and anxious) in contrast with those with normal trait anxiety, when exposed to threat-provoking stimuli at levels that were not consciously perceived.

In the people with high trait anxiety, unconscious information processing, when inaccessible to regulation by conscious processes, was very vulnerable to bias whose magnitude appeared to be determined by their level of trait anxiety, i.e. the greater the base level of anxiety, the greater the activation seen.

Many factors can cause overstimulation of the threat mechanisms, including chemical injury, bacterial, viral, or fungal infections, and emotional or psychological stress. When we are feeling threatened over a long period of time, our bodies learn to adapt to this unhealthy state, but at a large cost to our well being. Functions like rest, digestion, elimination, communication between cells, and reproduction are no longer viewed as essential and get overshadowed by our need for protection. This hypervigilant state takes up all of our energy, leaving little for day-to-day functioning. Over time, distorted and elevated sensory awareness becomes normal, and we may find ourselves more sensitive to everyday stimuli.

Patients who are undiagnosed slowly adapt to this state of poor health and change the way in which they live in order to accommodate the illness. Patients' survival and safeguarding of energy becomes a full-time job. They become shadows of their former selves. The brain and body adapt to this heightened level of threat and, over time, this inevitably changes their view of the world. Understandably patients become depressed. When forced to live in survival mode, their basic sense of trust in themselves, in others, and in the world feels shattered. No longer the happy-go-lucky people they once were, many turn into bitter pessimists. Happiness seems like a luxury that is only available to people who are still naïve about the world.

Slowly patients withdraw from society as their need for protection starts to dominate every aspect of their existence. If they reach out to those who offer help they often find themselves feeling disappointed and disillusioned – especially since the type of help they need is simply not available. This leads patients to question their ability to trust. Patients are left with a sense of helplessness and hopelessness – like they are invisible victims of a global war. Their attention is consumed with worry and a need to protect what little they have left of themselves.

This is what life is like for those who suffer from limbic system impairments. The cascading physical and emotional effects of an impaired threat mechanism are very real, and the suffering involved is horrendous. However, once the threat mechanisms are normalized again, the body can return to its natural state of growth and repair, allowing the patient to move forward in life again. This can seem quite miraculous, especially if a patient has been suffering over a long term. However, it is not a miracle in the sense that we do not know how this happens. Rather, the field of neuroplasticity is gradually gaining ground, and we are learning to use the inherent characteristics of the brain to reduce suffering.

WHY THE DYNAMIC NEURAL RETRAINING SYSTEM™ WORKS

DNRS is a self-directed program that helps patients decrease overactivated threat mechanisms in the brain, which normalizes sensory perception and regulates the overall stress response in the body. The techniques used in DNRS are based on neuroplasticity-based therapy, which encourages the brain to use dormant neural pathways or to build new neural pathways to restore normal function.

In medical terms, DNRS would be considered a top-down, neuroplasticity-based psychoneuroimmunological intervention.

It downgrades the brain's maladapted chronic stress response through rewiring limbic system circuits in the brain.

DNRS examines how trauma affects the stress mechanisms in the brain, how this expresses itself on physical, psychological, and emotional levels, and how all this affects overall health. DNRS helps patients move from a state of 'fight-or-flight' into a state of growth and repair where healing can take place. The program assists in altering the flood of stress biochemicals that activate cytokine activity and inflammation, effectively increasing energy and well-being and decreasing many symptoms of illness.

Let's take Susan as an example. Susan had moved into a new house that was recently renovated. New carpets, new paint, new everything. And while her new home looked aesthetically beautiful and might have been what many would consider a 'dream home', Susan was unknowingly immersed in a toxic stew. The high concentration of volatile organic compounds (VOCs) that were being released from the paint, carpets, and furniture were literally poisoning her brain and body. In fact, her cat died within five weeks of living in her new 'dream home.'

Susan's physical symptoms included headaches, body aches and pain, inability to focus or concentrate, poor memory, insomnia, food sensitivities, exhaustion, involuntary muscle twitching and weakness, heightened sense of smell and taste (especially for chemicals) and loss of voice with any degree of exposure to any sort of chemical.

Susan's initial trauma – the VOCs from her house – impaired her limbic system function and set into motion a brain trauma cycle. It activated an inflammatory response in her brain, which prompted a protective response that caused the brain's distorted perception of and reaction to a number of stimuli, and especially with any stimulus that was associated with the initial trauma.

The chemical injury from the toxic overload triggered a protective threat mechanism in Susan's brain. While her system was trying to cope with the toxins, other systems in her body were slowly giving way to more dominant, instinctual survival mechanisms. While her body was prioritizing the stress and survival functions like the overproduction of stress hormones which heighten sensory perception, it decreased her body's ability to process the toxins. In this state, many of the healthy systems of her body like cell growth and repair, immune system function, and detoxification were compromised, allowing the symptoms of illness to increase in scope and severity.

Soon she was unable to work or socialize with her friends, nor could she invite people into her home or go out to public places due to her severe reaction to chemicals. Going for a walk in her neighborhood became impossible due to dryer exhaust fumes. Given the impaired function of her limbic system, going into other people's homes wasn't possible either as common household chemicals would produce a life-threatening reaction in her system. Air fresheners, laundry soap, fabric softeners, cologne, perfume, deodorant, body lotions, cleaning products, new furniture, carpets, paint, and so on would cause a tailspin of symptoms that would leave her bedridden and cognitively impaired for days. The risk was just not worth it. Depression and anxiety soon set in, and understandably so when the world she was living in seemed uninhabitable. As is common with people who suffer from limbic system disorders, Susan slowly adapted her life to her illness. Fearing further exposures and consequent suffering, she started to live in isolation and avoidance. When she did experience an inadvertent exposure, on top of the physical reactions she would often find herself crying for no particular reason or responding with extreme anger and frustration. In addition to the physical symptoms, limbic system impairments also have an emotional component. When triggered, a range of inappropriate emotional reactions like sudden fits of rage, spontaneous crying, and sudden onset of severe depression are commonplace.

It took Susan five months to realize that it was indeed her home that was making her sick. And when she finally realized this, she moved out. However, by that time, the damage was already done. She was already suffering from toxic overload and brain trauma that affected her limbic system. The volatile organic compounds from new textiles, paints, and furniture had overwhelmed her system and resulted in trauma and subsequent cross wiring of neural circuits within the limbic system. Over time, the symptoms escalated, and Susan was literally starting to react to everything.

Susan's brain was so overloaded that it had lost the ability to discern between what was threatening and what was not. An impaired limbic system can fall prey to the process of 'priming,' where sensitivities spread easily from one stimulus to another – and in extreme cases sensitivities to the most essential things like food and water can develop.

During trauma, Susan's brain had unconsciously associated chemicals with extreme danger. Through repeated exposures and reactions, the neural circuits associated with this threat mechanism became hyperactivated and were set off by smaller and smaller amounts of chemicals. Her heightened sense of smell and taste, a symptom of her condition, caused her to perceive chemicals as life-threatening, at levels that most people cannot detect.

Her family doctor didn't know what she had or how to help her. She even tried various detoxification treatments and spent thousands of dollars on various supplements that were recommended by alternative health practitioners, yet she was still sick. Unfortunately, Susan's story is not uncommon.

Susan had difficulty finding a home where her body could actually rest. Eventually some friends of hers allowed her to stay in their wooden cabin located outside of the city. They removed all of the furniture and Susan lived in the empty cabin, except for an old mattress on the floor. Even the metal in the box spring and bed frame caused a reaction. She went from a thriving life to merely surviving in less than a year.

After attending the DNRS program, Susan noticed a shift in her sense of smell right away and a dramatic decrease in her symptoms and reactions within three days. However, it took her six months of dedicated practice to fully rewire her brain.

In order for Susan to change the unconscious protective patterns that were in play, she first had to understand how her brain was working and recognize what symptoms were part of the limbic system impairment.

All of us have habitual neural networks, that is, sequences and combinations of sequences of electrical impulses or highways of information that fire simultaneously on a regular basis. We have more neurons in our brains than stars in the universe and in any given moment there are over a million synapses firing in the average human brain. The brain is constantly playing an internal game of connect the dots, looking for patterns of association. For instance, if your mother or father wore a specific perfume or cologne habitually, when you smell that perfume or cologne out in the world, you are reminded of your mother or father. Once that association is established, information will travel that pathway faster and more easily. Information will always follow the path of least resistance. The more the pathway is used, the faster the information travels and the stronger the association. This is how all learning happens.

According to the "neurons that fire together – wire together" theory from Dr. Donald Hebb, the deeper the emotions associated with any given event, the stronger the neural networks become, and the faster the association and activation of the memory of the experience. This process happens so quickly and so automatically that patients may find themselves unconsciously reacting to a stimulus without consciously acknowledging an association or cause.

> *What most people don't know is that when they think about a highly charged emotional experience the brain will fire in the exact sequences and patterns as before; they are firing and wiring their brains to the past by reinforcing those circuits into evermore hard wired networks. They also duplicate the same chemicals in the brain and body (in varying degrees) as if they were experiencing the event again in that moment. Those chemicals begin to train the body to further memorize that emotion (Dispenza, 2012).*

With this process in mind, let us consider this same function with a limbic system impairment. Disorganization of neural networks in the limbic system causes a cross wiring of associations and skews perception. Once these circuits are impaired, specific thought patterns, emotional states, and behaviours actually become symptoms of dysfunction. Many of the thoughts, feelings, and behaviours are largely unconscious until we bring them to the surface of our awareness and start to discern if they are helpful or harmful. Again, 'protective' thoughts, feelings, and behaviours are not the fault of the patient. They are unconscious 'threat' reactions and are the result of limbic system trauma. Although they seem justifiable in the moment, they ultimately do not serve the recovery process. When these patterns are followed to their habitual conclusion, the patient inadvertently strengthens the pathological neural networks.

> *The way in which we learn and memorize information joins neurons together to form stronger connections by the*

'Law of Association'. ...When we are learning, we use past memories and prior experiences, things we already know (already wired synaptic connections), in order or build or project a new concept (Dispenza, 2007).

RECOGNIZING PATTERNS OF LIMBIC SYSTEM DYSFUNCTION

For Susan, recognizing which of her patterns were parts of the illness was an essential step in her recovery process. Recall there are a number of thoughts, emotions, behaviours, and physical symptoms that are telltale signs of a limbic system impairment. With a limbic system impairment, thought patterns generally tend toward the negative, such as reliving past traumas, or toward predicting future negative outcomes in any given situation. Some of the common emotions associated with limbic system trauma are feelings of fear, profound sadness, worry, hopelessness, shame, guilt, anger, inadequacy, remorse, powerlessness, resentment, and a state of hypervigilance. In addition, emotions are often exaggerated and inappropriate for the situation. Behavioural patterns are most often centred around avoidance of known triggers and result in the patient's isolation. In the case of chemical sensitivities, and electric hypersensitivity syndrome, the focus is on guarding health and preventing further reaction and suffering. For chronic fatigue and fibromyalgia sufferers, the focus of the protective behaviour is often about safeguarding energy expenditure and can also be in reaction to, or an attempt to prevent, physical pain. Heightened sensory perceptions including smell and taste (especially with MCS), touch (pressure sensitivity), hearing (loud sounds), seeing (light sensitivity), food sensitivities, and aversion response to chemical, electromagnetic, or other stimuli, characterize the physical symptoms along with non-specific pain, irregular body temperature, digestive issues, and inflammation.

THE BRAIN TRAUMA CYCLE

Before addressing our next topic, incremental training, let's briefly review the brain trauma cycle again. The initial trauma causes disorganization in limbic system circuits. This activates protective mechanisms and distorts sensory and stimulus perception. The protective mechanisms in the brain focus our attention on the perceived threat(s). The anterior cingulate cortex focuses the brain on the situation or offending stimulus. It then sends corresponding fear and threat messages to the amygdala, which activates the 'fight-or-flight' response. This activates the hypothalamus, which normally maintains a state of homeostasis. However, in a state of threat, the hypothalamus sends alert messages to the pituitary gland, which activates the adrenal glands (the HPA Axis) to release more stress hormones in order to maintain the heightened protective state.

This reaction in a short-term stress situation is actually beneficial, protecting us from threat and increasing physical abilities like strength, agility, and perception. However, in a limbic system trauma loop, this reaction feeds into itself, perpetuating the response and preventing the threat perception from receding.

The role of the hippocampus is to store information about the stimulus and to assign value and meaning for future protection. This is where the association gains strength and creates a faster neural pathway, making it easier for the brain to prepare for this particular threat. It is important to understand that this is an entirely unconscious protective response. Again, this may serve us well in a short-term situation, but in an impaired limbic system, this creates a well-worn path to a distorted stimulus response. Studies show neural dysfunction or neuronal loss in the hippocampus and the anterior cingulate gyrus in patients with PTSD, which contributes to limbic system dysfunction (Mahmutyazicioglu, K. Konuk, N., Atasoy, N., Atik, L., Gundogdu S, 2005).

Changing the neural circuits of the limbic system requires knowledge about how the brain works and the understanding that we can influence our brain so that, through our own free will, we can decrease symptoms associated with illness. Changing the brain through our own influence is known as self-directed neuroplasticity. However, as we know, change is not always easy and this process can take time.

In this regard, changing our beliefs about illness and altering associated protective behaviours can be very challenging. However, understanding why this change is necessary in the recovery process will assist in the continuous commitment that is needed in order to rewire neural circuits in the limbic system.

We need to keep in mind that during the initial trauma, the brain is overwhelmed or damaged. As such, the trauma itself is recorded in the neural circuits of the brain in a disorganized way. The resulting cross wiring becomes a subconscious pattern in the brain that gives rise to a constant state of 'fight-or-flight'.

This faulty wiring influences our state of physical health and well being, our emotional state, our thought patterns and alters our perception of safety. With repetition, these neural circuits have become the dominant pathway that the brain travels, making this pathway both stronger and faster. This unconscious pattern also influences our beliefs – what we hold to be true about ourselves and the world around us.

Where we choose to place our focus in any given moment will dictate how the brain works and can influence the recovery process. Staying stuck in patterns of a limbic system trauma loop keeps the brain and body in a constant state of 'fight-or-flight' which influences our natural healing abilities. Overriding these patterns allows our body to put its energy back into healing and repairing (a natural process that our bodies are designed to do).

Keep in mind that this is a real condition and the way to recover from brain trauma is through neuroplasticity.

Imperative to recovery is first recognizing and then interrupting the pathological patterns that are brought on by the malfunctioning protective mechanism. In understanding and treating the dysfunction, it is possible to influence the threat mechanism circuitry. The patient needs to learn detachment from the patterns and eventually replace them with healthier and more conscious responses. The new focus is to strengthen alternative pathways in the brain. This is known as 'top-down' modulation (direct regulation by the brain of physiological functions), where executive function (also known as cognitive control or supervisory attentional system), inhibits inappropriate amygdala hyperactivation.

Developing mindfulness of the habitual patterns that are associated with a limbic system trauma loop is essential in this process. As the patient steps into the 'curious observer' role, or what Dr. Schwartz calls the 'impartial observer,' they learn to develop a sense of curiosity about the situation. Rather than immediately reacting in old coping and protective habits that relate to symptoms of illness, the patient takes a step back and looks at the beliefs, thoughts, feelings, and physical symptoms that are associated with the reaction. By doing this, a patient is acting on the adage 'You are not what your brain is telling you'. A patient must realize that her brain is stuck in a fear and protective hiccup. The advice 'Don't believe everything you think, don't believe everything you feel and certainly do not believe every message that your body is sending you' is good to keep in mind when dealing with limbic system dysfunction, as the messenger is impaired.

Recognition of the various patterns of expression of limbic system dysfunction on physical, psychological, emotional, and behavioural levels is pivotal in order to change the deep wiring of the brain. Studies suggest that reappraisal, detachment, and distraction results in increased prefrontal activity (the area for higher learning like planning and decision making), an increase in anterior cingulate cortex activity (the region involved in attention and evaluation of emotional stimuli), and decreased amygdala activity (the structure involved in the fear response). The ability to change the brain through our conscious awareness is known as 'top-down regulation' (Modinos, G., Ormel, J. Aleman, A., 2010) (McRae, K., Hughes, B. Chopra, S. Gabrieli, J.D., Gross, J. J., Ochsner, K. N., 2010).

When a person has responded to a trigger and is in the middle of a reaction, employing executive function to overrule many of these instinctual reactions may seem counterintuitive, yet it is key to recovery. The seemingly 'instinctual' reactions are due to a protective mechanism gone awry. As we disengage from unconscious reactions, we are inhibiting the neural pathways that constantly overstimulate survival mechanisms in the limbic system. A considerable investment of time and commitment to the DNRS practice is necessary to cultivate a 'new normal' or to reinvent what makes up a patient's 'intuitive response'.

BECOMING AN ALCHEMIST

In order to interrupt a limbic system trauma loop, the patient will need to adopt new ways of thinking, feeling, and behaving. Creating a different understanding or perspective of the journey to date is an excellent way to alter brain pathways while empowering the patient to move forward. This requires that patients step into the role of alchemist in their life and begin to turn the 'negative' aspects of life into soul wisdom. From this sacred space of wisdom, they can choose to look at their lives from a different perspective. This change requires that they learn how to reframe their experiences and that they search for the lessons found within the journey. It is within this new perspective that the patient can move into a place of empowerment and positive change. This empowered position acts as the springboard to personal recovery and transformation.

This requires that the patient address stress in a different way. Research shows that how one thinks about stress will ultimately determine how beneficial or harmful it is. A recent study found that high amounts of stress and the perception that stress impacts health are each associated with poor health and mental health (Keller, A., Litzelman, K., Wisk, L.E., Maddox, T., Cheng, E.R., Creswell, P.D., Witt, W.P., 2012). In this light, developing techniques that change our perception of stress will help us manage stress more easily and ultimately have a more positive affect on health overall.

It is equally important to start to monitor and alter one's language in order to change habitual associations. Words are very meaningful and can trigger the brain to make associative connections that keep it stuck in a looping mechanism. It is important to be aware of language and conversational triggers that keep patients associated with illness. This is not an exercise in positive thinking or a form of denial. It is an exercise in rerouting the commonly traveled pathways that the brain has habitually taken.

THE MOMENT OF CHOICE

The brain is accustomed to travelling in specific patterns of neural networks that create a unique neurochemical cocktail. When patients change an understanding, a thought, an emotion or a behaviour, they use alternate neural networks or pathways and in doing so, change the neurochemical signature that is produced. In the beginning, this change feels uncomfortable because it is not familiar to the brain, and patients often encounter some resistance to this change. It is important that they not only recognize their own triggers and patterned reactions but that they also be aware that their unconscious and unique aversions to change stem from within the brain itself. In other words, the brain itself can be resistant to change. Within the DNRS program, these habitual and unconscious patterns are known as POPs, or 'pathways of the past.'

Recovery is not always a linear process and its course has its own ebb and flow. Every patient's recovery process is unique, and recovery times can vary greatly from patient to patient. Where some may see changes within a day or two, others may need weeks or months of dedicated practice. Patients must not get discouraged by the speed of their progress in comparison to others' progress, but should stay focused on their own dedication and on their own positive results. It is also important that patients avoid the urge to over-analyze their own process. Overanalyzing is akin to obsessing on the illness and keeps the brain in a looping mechanism, thus perpetuating the illness rather than circumventing it.

Similarly, symptoms of all limbic system conditions will manifest themselves distinctly for every individual. While suffering, a person finds it very difficult to believe that anyone else has suffered as much, has felt the same amount of pain, or has experienced the same level of exhaustion. This is an entirely understandable reaction given the amount of energy that has gone toward the illness and the accumulated pain and suffering. Patients will often experience a high level of frustration due to misdiagnosis or the inability of either the mainstream medical system or alternative health practices to diagnose or treat the illness effectively. Because of their past experience, the patients often come to believe that their condition is permanent or in some other way untreatable. Patients may also tend to think that their illness is worse, not as bad or different from others'. They may believe that the program could help someone else, in different circumstances, but that the program won't be effective for them. Although an amount of skepticism is normal, this reaction can be an expression of limbic system resistance to change. Although all the different conditions that are associated with limbic system impairment are unique, the recovery process is remarkably similar.

By the time a patient has found the DNRS program, they have likely been unsuccessfully treated by a number of different healthcare practitioners and have collected a large amount of information about potential causes for their illness. Out of necessity, many patients have, in fact, become experts of their own bodies and of their own illnesses. However, the nature of neuroplasticity is so different from other models of treatment that the collected information may actually act as an obstacle to recovery in the DNRS program. Success with this program requires that the patient learn how to work within a neuroplasticity model, which often involves setting aside more traditional medical ideas.

For example, we have been taught to believe that pain is the body's way of telling us that something is wrong – which ordinarily would be a perfectly logical idea. However, what we fail to recognize in this belief is that the brain is capable of sending faulty messages to the body, expressed as pain and discomfort. As we have seen, some forms of pain can actually be signs of limbic system dysfunction. When the root of the problem is in the disorganization of neural circuits, it becomes ineffective to chase symptoms.

Because pain is associated with so many different limbic system-associated illnesses, patients often find themselves obsessively focused on pain. As a result, patients will constantly mentally check their bodies to track, alleviate, or prevent symptoms.

Although it is a rational and protective response, this belief system about pain and discomfort leads to limiting behaviours. Over time and through repetition, the limiting pattern is strengthened and reinforces a limbic system loop. In order for the patient to successfully rewire the limbic system, they need to recognize the messages as false and expand their ability to visualize and actualize positive outcomes. Gradually they move beyond their perceived expectations of the past.

A typical sign of limbic system dysfunction is to revisit negative experiences or traumatic events, replaying the situation in the imagination repetitively and seemingly without resolution or end. The revisited trauma continuously activates negative thoughts and emotions that perpetuate and strengthen the trauma pathways in the brain. Similarly, a patient may find herself caught in a loop of negative thought patterns, negative self-dialogue, or anticipation of negative outcomes.

Another sign of limbic system impairment that is not commonly thought of as a symptom of illness is erratic mood swings. Because the limbic system is at the base of our emotional well-being, this actually makes good sense. An imbalance in the limbic system will logically have an effect on our emotional responses. When triggered, a patient may experience extreme negative emotions such as explosive rage, sudden and profound sadness, and/or repetitive suicidal thoughts. These thoughts and emotions can seem justified in the context of the illness; however, they are recognized as signs of dysfunction when interpreted by the patient as exaggerated and/or inappropriate to the situation. Also, a patient can experience an inappropriate physiological response to an exposure that is typically interpreted as 'emotional,' such as spontaneous and uncontrollable crying. Depression and increased emotional sensitivity are associated with low serotonin levels, which are common in limbic system dysfunction conditions.

There are many ways to increase serotonin in the brain without drugs. It is common knowledge that exercise and bright light can assist with increasing serotonin levels. What is not so well known is that self-induced changes in mood can also change serotonin levels, such as revisiting a happy memory (Perreau-Linck E, Beauregard M, Gravel P, Paquette V, Soucy JP, Diksic M, Benkelfat C, 2007). However, the ability to access positive memories or positive emotional states can be challenging for the patient suffering from limbic system dysfunction. Some good starting points to cue the brain's memory of happy events is to ask friends and family members for positive stories, look at photographs, or watch funny videos on the internet. This might feel unnatural at first; however, with practice the brain relearns how to access positive memories and emotions. This process requires a degree of emotional awareness as we learn not to entertain negative thoughts and feelings.

It often does not 'feel right' to engage in different thoughts, feelings, and behaviours as this change does not feed the habitual neural circuits that perpetuate the loop. This action is taking attention away from a familiar routine and can feel like a form of loss. Such a reaction speaks to how important it is for patients to embrace the new beliefs about themselves and their condition. Patients cannot believe that their chronic illness will continue and embrace change simultaneously. The old beliefs only start to change when patients start to experience shifts in their illness. However, in order to experience this shift, they need to commit wholeheartedly to the practice. The limbic system responds like a three-year-old child. It tends to react without consciously evaluating incoming sensory information. It is up to the patient to employ executive function and to override the habitual limbic reactions with healthier reasoning and responses.

The ability to change our emotional state, even when threat mechanisms in the limbic system are firing, requires that we think beyond the symptoms in the moment. This gets easier with focused and consistent repetition. The focus shifts from symptoms to strengthening alternate brain circuitry. When the threat response is sufficiently dampened and the new circuitry is strong enough, the symptoms will naturally start to dissipate.

During the rewiring process, it is very important for patients to consistently acknowledge the success that has been reached; the reminder of past successes serves as motivation to stay focused on their accomplishments in moments of weakness. A trigger moment may temporarily cause patients to lose sight of the gains they have made. However, the skills they have developed will allow them to recover from a trigger situation more rapidly.

At times, because the symptoms are physical in nature, patients may feel as though they have no conscious control over their body. Therefore, they will likely feel justified in returning to their habitual coping behaviours. However, this is counterproductive to recovery. While having a home that is completely environmentally healthy is a great strategy for anyone, we must keep in mind that in the case of limbic system dysfunction, the brain can be picking up on minute levels of stimuli as life threatening. Repetition of the strategies for rewiring limbic system function will create new neural circuits and eventually establish a 'new normal,' opening the mind to a whole new world of possibilities. Once a shift takes place, it becomes easier for a patient to be in different environments, and to have more positive thoughts, as the brain is less entrenched in a survival state of fear, worry, and anxiety. It is not uncommon for patients to notice that the cloud of depression that accompanied their illness has simply evaporated, allowing them access to positive emotional states again.

Blame centred thoughts and behaviours can lead to a negative focus and can detract from the recovery process. It is understandable that someone who has acquired MCS through chemical exposure would react with a desire to hold the responsible party accountable. Beyond that, a wish to rid the world of this chemical in order to prevent anyone else from exposure and potential illness is perfectly rational. Although this is a noble endeavour, focusing on this while engaged in the recovery process is not a productive use of energy and can impede the recovery process. Patients can return to their advocacy efforts once the recovery process is complete. Besides, they will likely have considerably more energy for such activism at that time. Furthermore, the act of blaming can extend to any number of people, circumstances, and situations that patients feel is holding back their progress in some way. Instead, it is important for patients to focus on their own recovery and their own ability to heal for the duration of the recovery process.

INCREMENTAL TRAINING

Attending a live DNRS program or purchasing the instructional DVD program with individual coaching is strongly recommended to gain more clarity about the rewiring process before attempting any type of incremental training. Rewiring the limbic system is not an intellectual process, but rather an experiential one that is best done with initial supervision and the opportunity to fully immerse oneself in 'neuroplasticity bootcamp'.

Incremental training is a form of 'shaping' which Dr. Edward Taub describes in the use of constraint induced therapy with stroke patients. In the case of limbic system rehabilitation, incremental training involves awareness of established patterns and challenging the brain with progressively more intense triggers over time. This process requires compassion and a willingness to let go of beliefs and behaviours that may have served as a protective device. These beliefs and behaviours may have served the patient well in the past; however, they can act as barriers to success if held too rigorously.

When the brain is in a heightened neuroplastic state (e.g. in response to a trigger), it is capable of the greatest change. The trigger heightens the neural pathways involved with the fear network and allows change in the neural pathways to occur more easily. When rewiring the limbic system, this is a desirable state. Research suggests that combinations of exposure therapy, response prevention strategies, and cognitive behaviour therapy can decrease amygdala hyperreactivity and normalize anterior cingulate cortex activity (Shum,F.W, Wu, Lo, Zhao, M. Yoyoda, H., Xu, H, Ren, M., Ren, M. Pinaud, R. Ko, S., Lee, Y. Daang, B., Zhou, M., 2007). One must keep in mind that over challenging may cause distress and therefore, it is important to find balance between challenging the brain and overdoing it. This balance is different for each person and will change over time as the patient's limbic system changes and the training zone expands.

NEUROPLASTICITY WORKING FOR YOU

It is important to bear in mind that the 'fires together – wires together' theory also applies to positively charged experiences. When a patient focuses attention on a positive emotion, they strengthen the positive association and its related biochemistry, which can assist greatly in recovery. Thus, repetition is essential to recovery, as it takes time for a patient to establish normalized and healthy neural pathways.

NECESSARY SELF-AWARENESS

For the DNRS program to be successful, it is imperative that a patient be able to step into the role of the 'curious observer.' The recognition of personal neural patterns and the necessity to interrupt them is key to rerouting the dysfunctional brain patterns. The ability to recognize unique dysfunctional patterns represents the first step in rewiring the limbic system. The ability to be the observer will help patients to distance themselves emotionally and assist them in thinking, feeling, and behaving in ways that are greater than their reactions or symptoms. Rewiring limbic system function can be akin to defying gravity as the patient learns to discern the signals from the brain and question the nature of their illness. Part of this process involves questioning emotional threat cues. As I noted earlier, the limbic system is emotionally like a three-year-old and is looking for both verbal cues (e.g. talking about symptoms) and nonverbal cues (e.g. body language). When compromised, the limbic system is constantly searching for evidence to support a 'fight-or-flight' state. Just as you would parent a three-year-old child, it is very important that healthy behaviour boundaries and consistent instruction are approached in a loving and nurturing way to healing your limbic system. With discipline and repetition, the limbic system will follow conscious guidance and be lead into a healthy and relaxed state.

IS DNRS A GOOD FIT FOR ME?

While the DNRS program has guided many successful recoveries, there are circumstances where a patient may not be a good candidate for the program, e.g. if a patient is experiencing an extreme level of stress such as ending a relationship, the recent loss of a parent or life partner, a change in residence, or the tragedy of homelessness, or if the patient is experiencing a significant health condition like cancer, stroke, or a serious heart condition. Although it may still be possible to rewire limbic system function within these circumstances, the added stress can represent additional challenges in this process. And while a number of mental health issues may be helped by the program, such as anxiety, depression, post-traumatic stress disorder, and obsessive compulsive disorder, there are some conditions that can make the program extremely difficult and can affect a patient's success. These include bipolar disorder, attention deficit hyperactivity disorder, dementia, schizophrenia, or other personality disorders. Other conditions that may affect success with the program are significant brain or head trauma, and any drug or alcohol addictions.

These circumstances can impact a patient's ability to concentrate and to dedicate themselves to the practice of the DNRS program which is essential to success. A patient must be committed to practice, with boot camp discipline. Patients can also benefit from taking advantage of the extra services offered by DNRS, such as the community forum, teleconferences, and individual coaching sessions with certified DNRS Coaches.

CHAPTER 7

Allergic to Everything

Racheal Stanley was 34 years old and in the prime of her life when she started to develop symptoms of environmental illness. Racheal was happily married to her husband Curtis, and collectively they had 6 children ranging in ages from nine to eighteen years old. To meet the needs of their combined family, they moved into their new home in Dallas, Texas in September of 2007.

It wasn't until 2009 that Racheal started to notice symptoms. At that time, she did not link the symptoms to her home, nor did she know that the symptoms that she was experiencing were related to environmental illness – that particular diagnosis did not come until years later.

Initially Racheal suffered from flu-like symptoms that included overall aches and body pain, headaches, overwhelming fatigue, and difficulty sleeping. The pain eventually became relentless, and Racheal began to experience a lot of back and spine pain that was unexplainable. Over the course of a few months, they bought six different bed mattresses, thinking that perhaps a better bed would help to alleviate the pain, but this did not help. In fact, in retrospect both Racheal and her husband Curtis realized that bringing new furniture into their home that was loaded with toxic chemicals, was absolutely the worst thing they could do. They didn't realize that the chemicals off-gassing from the mattresses were a factor in making her condition worse.

Racheal's symptoms escalated to include depression along with extreme anxiety – a deadly combination. Over time, Racheal noticed that she was getting anxious about everything. She also started having severe panic attacks. As long as Racheal can remember, she had always had claustrophobia, along with a fear of flying and of being in elevators, and as her health continued to decline, the panic attacks and claustrophobia worsened as well.

Racheal also noticed that she had gained weight for no apparent reason, and no matter how much she exercised, the weight just simply would not come off.

In 2009, Racheal started to experience heart problems. In Racheal's own words:

> The first time, I believe, was in 2009, it was the summer, we were on a vacation in San Antonio for our anniversary, and I started having a skipping heart beat. We could literally feel it skip every third or fourth beat, so we went to a cardiologist and they did the test where you wear a heart monitor for 24 hours. When I went back to the heart doctor, he said I was having 3,400 PVC's (premature ventricular contractions) a day which is the most he'd ever seen on a heart monitor, but he couldn't tell me why and couldn't explain it and just said it sometimes happens. Almost one-third of my heart beats were irregular. The skipping would settle down for a while but they always came back.

Racheal was also suffering from gastrointestinal symptoms like digestive issues, bloating, and nausea. She had been experiencing stomach problems for a couple of years. She also had multiple cysts on her ovaries and was frequently in pain.

Additionally, she constantly felt like she had a urinary tract infection and had been to see ten different doctors for that symptom alone. Although all of the tests came back negative, the symptoms persisted.

Racheal also began to exhibit neurological symptoms. She went to numerous doctors trying to diagnose the cause of the tingling in her fingers, her feet, and her toes. She also experienced muscle twitching and flinching that would keep her awake at night. Racheal says:

> I kept waking up with extremities that felt like they were asleep or they were burning, so I would see a neurologist, and they would do MRIs and of course not find anything. But there was always the "maybe you have MS" or different diagnoses they would throw out there, but they could never confirm them. My balance was also very poor. I couldn't even stand at church – we would go to church, and I'd bow my head to pray and close my eyes, and I'd fall over.

In addition to the growing list of symptoms, signs of cognitive impairment were also apparent. As Racheal describes it:

> I remember sometimes being at stoplights, going from all of these multiple doctors, and I would get confused and scared and not know which way I was going or where I was at, or how I got there. I remember calling my husband and saying, 'I'm really scared – I don't know where I'm at.' I would just zone out a lot. Total brain fog. I couldn't remember names, I couldn't remember appointments, and sometimes I even couldn't remember family names. So definitely lots of memory problems. I also couldn't do simple math or remember how to spell words.

A feeling of "fullness" or "pressure" in her head was also a major symptom. Racheal says:

> I had a lot of fullness and pressure, and I remember waking up and it felt kind of like I had pins and needles in my head, a kind of tingling at the top and the base of my head. That feeling of fullness was so extreme that it felt like my head was going to blow off all the time – just like it could explode because it was so full of pressure.

Racheal noticed that some of her senses had heightened. If she was around even the smallest amount of chemical or scented products, she could smell and taste them from a long distance away. If someone had laundered their clothing in scented laundry soap and fabric softener, Racheal could smell and taste a very sharp, bitter, and toxic quality.

Racheal describes the first time she noticed that her sense of smell had really changed. Racheal told me:

> The kids got in the car one day with a big rubber ball, and when they did I became very nauseous and had a headache, and that was when I first started noticing that I was super-sensitive to smell. This also escalated to include dryer sheets and perfumes and just about everything.

Prior to this, Racheal had also developed other sensitivities that seemed unrelated at the time. She noticed that she had become extremely sensitive to noise. You can imagine how challenging this might be with six children! Often this was too much for Racheal to endure. Racheal goes on to explain:

> *I literally crawled into a ball and stayed in my bedroom*
> *– especially when my kids got home. I couldn't tolerate the*
> *sound of them playing or bouncing balls or the constant*
> *level of noise. I had to be very secluded.*

Bright lights were also bothering her. Direct sunlight, the lights in doctors' offices, and car headlights while driving at night would hurt her eyes.

Racheal also developed electric hypersensitivity syndrome (EHS) but did not know what it was. She describes the strange sensations that accompany this illness:

> *I didn't know that's what it was, but probably six months*
> *to a year before February of 2011, I would notice that I'd*
> *be sitting on the couch, and I would feel like a vibration in*
> *my leg or my foot, and I would start looking for my cell*
> *phone because it felt like I was sitting on a cell phone. But*
> *there wouldn't be a phone there. There may be one going*
> *off in another room, but I was picking up on it sitting on*
> *the couch. I know it sounds crazy, but I could.*

As the illness continued to worsen, she developed severe insomnia and, at one point, she did not sleep for days at a time. As a result, her nervous system became exhausted, and her anxiety and depression increased. She noticed that she no longer enjoyed things that previously brought her joy. She had become extremely anxious about social situations, which was highly unlike her. Racheal describes this horrific time in her life:

> *It was November, 2010, and I guess my nervous system*
> *was in such a heightened state that I would be up for days –*

I couldn't settle down enough to even sleep and would just walk the house. I even had panic attacks. Curtis couldn't go to work for weeks. He had to sit with me, and I literally just shook. I sat in a ball and shook with anxiety. I wasn't even able to sit in a room with my kids any more. I mean they had to knock on the door and were scared to come in because Mom was curled up shaking in a ball. I didn't want for them to see me like that. And I didn't want to do that to them. My husband had to spend so much time taking care of me that he was losing his company and his business, and he couldn't work, and he was sick with worry.

Needless to say, Racheal's illness was difficult for the entire family. No one knew what was happening, and they all felt very helpless as they stood by and watched their mother deteriorate.

There were times when Racheal thought that the best option would be death. Not that she wanted to end her life – she just wanted the suffering to end. At times, this seemed like the only logical answer:

It was so bad and I just didn't want to live that way. I didn't want to live in pain. I didn't know what was wrong with me. I had a tingling in my head and my feet and everywhere I hurt. I was tired. I was starting to hallucinate because I didn't sleep for days because I couldn't settle down.

Of course, by this time Racheal was extremely depressed and feeling hopeless, and suicidal thoughts became commonplace. She went on to describe the day that she almost followed through with it:

There was one particular day that I remember clearly. I was so depressed and so anxious – and I had a psychiatrist who was trying me on every drug possible to try to settle down whatever was going on with my body. I remember lying in the bathtub and going under the water and thinking, 'I don't even want to come up from this bathtub because I don't think I can do this any more. If this is how life's going to be, I can't do it.' And I remember looking up as I was starting to lose consciousness, and I saw little Gavin's picture [Racheal's youngest son] sitting on the sink in my bathroom and managed to pull myself out of the water and called Curtis.

Through my tears I told him what had happened and how I was feeling. He immediately came home from work, and we hugged and cried and sat on the floor. It was probably the darkest time of my life.

It's hard to understand but when your body's doing crazy stuff and you can't understand it, and nobody else understands it, and you're not yourself and you're miserable and you're thinking crazy thoughts and your body's doing crazy things, it's hard to have hope.

Eventually Racheal ended up seeing an environmental doctor in Dallas, Texas in 2011. They did a battery of tests on Racheal's home where they found black mould and high levels of formaldehyde. She was informed that her house was not a healthy place and that she could not recover in the home due to severe mould toxicity. Racheal knew she was getting sick, but this was the first time anyone had identified the house as the source of the problem. Racheal describes her initial experience with the environmental doctor this way:

I really did not know what was wrong with me until I saw the environmental doctor in Dallas, Texas in 2011. Little did I know that the room that I secluded myself in was actually making everything worse. There was black mould in the room, and it was also off-gassing all kinds of chemicals from the painting and staining that were just done. I was exposed all day and all night.

The environmental doctor did a barrage of testing, and then I found out I was allergic to everything. I was allergic to every food, every chemical, and pretty much everything around me. My body was just in a super-heightened sense of 'fight-or-flight' – it was like I was allergic to everything. Yes, I was allergic to every mould, every tree, every pollen, and every grass. Pretty much anything I tested for – cotton and every fabric. Just everything you could imagine. Of course, they tested our home, and we did have the black mould toxins. So they did that testing, and my body showed mycotoxins associated with the black mould and very high levels of heavy metals. My immune system was just crashed. My T-cells were very low so I wasn't able to fight things off. Pretty much everything that could be off was off. I was also diagnosed with Crohn's disease.

Racheal was advised to move into a sterile environment, away from her family while receiving treatments from her environmental doctor, in the hopes that this would assist with her recovery. Racheal moved in to a single room in a complex with others who were suffering from similar environmental illnesses. Her room was completely tiled and minimally furnished. She had a wood frame futon to ensure that her bed did not contain any of the metal that she was reacting to at the time. Some people who were living there had been there for years.

This complex was considered to be one of the few 'safe' places to live for many who suffer from environmental illness. Here's how Racheal describes her situation:

> It was cold, it was white, it was sterile, it was depressing, it was lonely. I watched multiple people come in and out that were very, very sick. I watched people go into seizures in rooms next to me. I watched a man rolled out on a gurney dying of a heart attack and then pretty much died in front of us one night. It was a very, very dark time. It was very depressing. It was very cold. It was very sterile.

As you can well imagine, Racheal was devastated to have to leave her husband and children. Living in the sterile room surrounded by other patients was a constant reminder of what her life had become. Needless to say, this was extremely distressing for her entire family. Moving to the complex was a desperate attempt to get better, but by that point, they were willing to do anything.

Her husband and children would visit Racheal when they could, but Curtis would have to change his clothes beforehand because the smell of his work clothes would make Racheal sick. Often her children couldn't even go into the room to see their mother because they had unknowingly picked up some kind of chemical or scent during their journey to see her. Perhaps they were around someone who had used dryer sheets or someone who had been wearing perfume or cologne. The chemicals would stick to their clothing, thereby contaminating them and making it unsafe for Racheal to see them. It was heart-breaking for everyone. Racheal explains:

If my kids went to a friend's house and came and visited me, I couldn't have them around me because maybe they were around somebody with a dryer sheet or around somebody with perfume or maybe they smelled like rubber or tires on cars.

Meanwhile, the escalating costs for Racheal's medical treatments were breaking the bank. While trying to care for his ailing wife, Curtis had to hire a CEO to run his company as he was completely enmeshed in trying to take care of Racheal and their six children. Unfortunately, the CEO he hired took advantage of his extremely fragile situation and ended up stealing money from the company. Curtis was beside himself and devastated both emotionally and financially. This was the last straw. Completely shattered, Curtis even wondered if his own death might be helpful. At least the life insurance policy would help with Racheal's medical bills and the children. The stress was almost too much for him to handle.

Of course, this experience had a profound affect on their children. Racheal goes on to explain:

It was hard. Gavin, he was little, and he developed a lot of fears, he and some of our other children became scared of electricity and smells because they didn't want to be sick too. They became very paranoid and scared. It was hard on my daughter – she didn't have a mom and had to do a lot on her own and she was very lonely and very scared with her mother being sick. My then 15-year-old son, he turned to drugs. He was very scared, and I had been his stability. Curtis was with me a lot and our son was very lonely. He has since been in treatment for drugs twice and still battles with addiction that started during that time. Curtis's sons, well, they fell apart. Prior to me being sick, they had their Dad with them and now he was with me all the time, and that caused a lot of problems. We had to go through some therapy because they felt like they were abandoned, and it was hard on the family as a whole. It was hard on our marriage because Curtis had to work to pay for all these costs, and then he had to take care of kids, but I was very sick and I felt like I needed him, and I felt isolated, so that caused problems. So it was a hard time for everybody.

Racheal's symptoms continued to worsen, especially after having an electro-current treatment for back pain:

They tried to do some electro-current treatment for my back but because of the treatment, my body just went into total shaking, and I would almost say like little baby seizures, where I just shook uncontrollably. After that, even if I was standing near a light I could feel an electrical current in my foot. It was pretty crazy.

She goes on to say:

It was just a very, very dark, long time. I was away from my kids for a long time. It was very hard on them, and it was hard on my husband. I had family that thought I had a psychiatric illness, I had friends that no longer were my friends because this was just too crazy to even comprehend, so I was very alone. Curtis and the kids would come see me when they could, but he was trying to be Dad and run a business and make money to pay the outrageous costs that we were paying for treatment. I was being told each day that there was something new that I was allergic to, so I pretty much just created this bubble in the room and never felt safe leaving it. So it was eight months of being there, and once again, I got to the point where I didn't want to live that way. I mean, when it became evident that I was not getting better, I would entertain some really desperate thoughts like 'oh, I need to move to the desert where there's nothing that I will react to'. It just became so crazy. I knew that there had to be something else because the treatments that I was undergoing or had already done, whether it was hyperbaric or sauna or vitamin C, or outrageous nutrient IVs that cost hundreds of thousands of dollars was not helping.

With his wife tenuously clinging to life, Curtis was constantly researching on the internet trying to find answers. During one of his visits to Racheal, Curtis came upon the Dynamic Neural Retraining System website. Immediately, he printed out everything on the website and laid it out on the floor for Racheal because, with her EMF sensitivities, Racheal couldn't be near the computer.

He wept as he read it to her and said, "You know, Babe, I think this is it – I *know* it is". With conviction in his voice, Curtis continued, "I know this is what's going to get you well and we'll do whatever we have to do to have you meet Annie Hopper and take this program. This is what's going to change our lives!" Racheal relayed this story to me in a matter of fact tone and continued by saying:

And so that's kind of how it happened. My youngest son Gavin had overheard the conversation, and he was excited, and he knew that there was somebody that was *coming from Canada that was going to get his Mom well. He was very hopeful and not for a second did he have a doubt that it wasn't going to work. So he was really excited. Of course, I was very skeptical because there was so many things we'd done and tried and they just weren't working. I knew it sounded really good, but I didn't really know what it consisted of yet. I was very skeptical. I had already spent over $300,000 looking for an answer and nobody could help me. So I think a certain amount of skepticism is normal. But when somebody's operating with a limbic system dysfunction, it's really hard to get them to think that anything's going to work. The illness was also making me more paranoid and more negative, so when you're like that, it's hard to believe that anything is good.*

Racheal attended the DNRS program in December 2011 when I travelled to Dallas and facilitated the program in one of the small sterile hotel rooms at the complex where Racheal had been living isolated from her family. Everyone who attended the program had some degree of chemical sensitivities, so it was extremely important that no one in the room had any scents or chemicals on their clothing or in the personal hygiene products that they used. Everyone was sent a list months in advance to ensure that the space would be as safe as possible.

At the time of the program, Racheal had just recently moved into a new house to be with her family. Although she was still very sick, she decided to leave the complex to live with her family again. While Racheal had been living at the complex, Curtis had ensured that all of the remediation work on their home was done to make the house safe again. Although their house was then considered safe, the doctors thought it would not be healthy either psychologically or emotionally for Racheal to go back. So,

Curtis and Racheal sold their old home and bought a new one. The entire family still had to obey very strict guidelines in order for Racheal to be at home with them: no chemicals, no scents, no electronics, no cell phones, etc. Although Racheal was still very sick, the ability to be at home with her family again was emotionally and psychologically the best thing to do.

It was shortly after Racheal moved back home again that I spoke to her on the phone. The first thing that stood out for me was her endearing Texan accent and how she referred to me as "Ma'am." She was excited about attending the upcoming program in Dallas. Although she was still skeptical, the science behind the program made sense to her.

When Racheal began the program, she started to notice some changes in psychological and emotional symptoms almost right away. With her new understanding about how the toxic injury had affected her brain, she immediately felt less anxious and even hopeful. She wasn't as worried about her heightened sense of smell and no longer took it as a 'warning' sign of something toxic in her environment but understood on a fundamental level that her sensory perception was distorted because of limbic system dysfunction, and that this was triggering a faulty alarm message that was affecting many systems in her body. Over the course of the next few days, Racheal noticed that her sense of smell started to normalize.

That was all the evidence she needed in order to know that the DNRS program was the answer that they had been searching and praying for.

Racheal was so excited that she shared this great news with her family and enthusiastically talked about all of the things that she would soon be able to do. She explained to her husband and children what she was learning about her brain and relayed some guidelines to them about how they could help her in her recovery process.

They all had a renewed sense of hope and faith that Racheal would soon be well again – especially Gavin, her youngest son.

Within a week of attending the program, Racheal went to a restaurant that she hadn't been to in a couple of years. She excitedly recalls that time:

> *Five days after completing the program there was a birthday dinner and my grandfather came. I hadn't seen him in a couple of years, and we cried because we were so thrilled to see each other. It was almost unbelievable; there I was, in a steakhouse with my Granddad. The restaurant had propane gas and was full of people. There was lots of noise and lots of smells. But nothing bothered me! I ate fried food and I ate ranch dressing. I ate things that were things that I had been told I was allergic to, and I sat and did great at the restaurant. And then we followed my Granddad to his hotel, which was full of chemicals from hotel cleaning stuff and smelled of chlorine from an outdoor pool, but it didn't smell bad! I was able to sit in his room and visit with him. When we got back in the car to go home, Curtis and I were overjoyed and almost in shock. I was able to do all of this, and only 5 days later.*

Racheal goes on to explain that, even though she was able to do lots of things that she was unable to do before, she was not fully recovered and was still experiencing various symptoms:

> *I mean, I wasn't completely recovered at that point. I still struggled with things, and there were times that I'd have to do the exercises more than an hour a day. But five months later, I went on a girls' weekend trip in the hill country in Texas and floated down the river. I was staying with a bunch of smelly,*

perfumed up girls in a condo and floating on the river. I would
say that I was 80% recovered by then. A year after taking
the program, we took a trip to Florida and stayed in a regular
hotel. That's when I knew that I was 100% recovered.

When I inquired as to how Racheal lives her life now in
terms of environmental awareness, her response was:

> *We live, I think, with environmental awareness. We*
> *don't use pesticides or use paint with lots of VOCs. We don't*
> *introduce a lot of chemicals, but we don't go overboard either.*
> *I think we're kind of moderate. I don't use fabric softener,*
> *and I don't use detergents that are scented. But my shampoo*
> *and conditioner do have scent, and they smell really good.*
> *We try to eat organic, but not everything is organic. ... I*
> *don't make my kids change their clothes when they come*
> *through the door. My kids wear scented products ... and I*
> *don't notice those things anymore. ... I mean, I eat fast food,*
> *I go to the gym, I get in the sauna... just to make me feel*
> *good, but not because I'm thinking, 'I'm detoxing.' I like to*
> *work out. I like to be healthy and make healthy choices but I*
> *eat cake, I eat anything I want to. We try to be environmen-*
> *tally smart, but we don't take it to extremes where we are*
> *stressed out about it or obsessed about it.*

For Racheal, the entire experience of having had environmental illness is something that she would much rather forget.
She goes on to say:

> *Curtis and I couldn't even drive by that complex with-*
> *out breaking into tears. I mean, for the first year or two.*
> *Even now when we drive by on the freeway, we won't look*

that direction because we don't want to remember it. It was a dark time. We are still very sad for those who are still suffering, and I'd love to share the good news with those people but a lot of them, for whatever reason, don't want to hear it.

Prior to attending the DNRS, Racheal had been to approximately 20 specialists and had spent over $300,000 searching for answers.

What is important to note is that Racheal did not undergo any chelation treatments to detoxify heavy metals from her body. Racheal spoke to this when she said:

> The doctors at the environmental clinic said that my body wasn't strong enough to handle that because I guess some of the lab levels were pretty poor. I know that my T-cells and my immunoglobulin and so forth were extremely low, so they just thought that I wouldn't be able to tolerate that.

When I asked if she had ever had any kind of heavy metal detoxification treatment to date she replied:

> No, ma'am, but oddly enough I just recently saw a naturopath just for hormonal stuff, and I don't have a thyroid, so she was just kind of checking normal stuff. And she did check for metals just to see where we were at, and I had no metals, so somehow, at some point, anything that was in me that was metals is gone. And something else I wanted to tell you is that I went back to my female doctor for an exam, and I had zero cysts on my ovaries. Like, they were all gone, and she couldn't explain that.

When I asked Racheal what she would like to say to all of the doctors that she had previously seen she said:

> *I would pray for them also that they would learn more about what you're teaching and that this is a dysfunction... I don't know if dysfunction is the correct word... in the brain. It is trauma to the brain. It is a limbic system cross wiring. I just wish they would not scare people so bad. I know for me they made it very, very scary and seem very overwhelming. I think living in that fear causes people to feel desperate. I think it makes them suicidal. I think it makes them feel hopeless. I wish that they knew more about what you did because I think the illness could be eliminated to a very, very small percent if they were treating it correctly. I don't know that they grasp it. I know that since I did your program, my immune system now is fabulous, and when the rest of my family this winter got the flu or stomach bugs, I don't get the flu, I don't get stomach bugs, I don't get sick anymore. So, I don't know. I wish they understood what you're teaching.*

When I asked Racheal what she would say to other people who are still suffering she said:

> *I would tell them that your program is a life saver. We even gave the DVD to our son in college because he was suffering from anxiety, it's helped him a lot, in fact it even helped his golf game. It's also helped our youngest son Gavin. He was having nightmares and fear that people were poisoning him, and he worried all the time. So the program also worked for him, and he doesn't worry anymore. So, I think it can be life changing for everyone. It*

even worked on fears and anxiety that I had before I was diagnosed with environmental illness. I wouldn't get on elevators, I wouldn't go in closed, dark spaces, and I didn't like to fly. Well, this last week I flew for the first time in six or seven years and did amazing. We stayed on the 59th floor of a hotel and I don't even flinch when I get in an elevator anymore, so it's life changing.

I mean, it truly changes your brain, and I would've not known that before. It's freed me in ways beyond the illness. I'd had some post-traumatic stuff and I think that added to my condition – you know, years of abuse and neglect and abandonment and just worry. I think I had been in a 'fight-or-flight' state since the age of five. So it broke a lot of years of looping of just bad stuff. So I would just tell them it's life changing. If you want out of MCS or EMF or fibromyalgia, depression, then this is the cure. The answer is in changing the brain.

At the end of the program, Curtis and Gavin came in to pick up Racheal and take her home. When they entered the room, Curtis immediately came over to express his heartfelt thanks to me and turned to Gavin, as if to say, "it's your turn now, buddy." Gavin had obviously just woken up from a nap and was still wiping the sleep from his eyes. He looked up at me and said, "This is for you." He was holding a small gift bag and reached up to give it to me. I leaned down to meet him and said "thank you, that was very thoughtful of you." I was very moved by his generosity and thoughtfulness, but was not prepared for what was inside the bag. As I looked inside the bag, I noticed there were small presents, along with a card. It was a hand-written "thank-you" card that Gavin had made. The picture on the front of the card had two big red and orange crayon hearts with

THANKS printed in big letters across the page. I could feel a big lump in my throat and tears escape from my eyes as I continued to read the priceless words inside. It said:

> Hi, I'm Gavin.
>
> Thank you for heeling my Mom.
> I can't wait for her to be better so she can run and play with me. I am eight years old. I like to play football and baseball.
> I am number eleven and fifteen.
> I hope you make my Mom feel all better.
> My Mom and Dad have been talking about all the trips they want to go on and how good you are and the best docter.
>
> Thank you for heeling my Mom.
> Love, Gavin.

As hard as I tried, I could not contain my tears, and they happily flowed down my cheeks. As I hugged them all goodbye, I felt a pure sense of happiness. Not only for Racheal and her family, but also for all the lives they will touch because of her recovery. Furthermore, I knew that this was just the beginning of her second chance at life.

I've framed Gavin's letter, and it hangs on my office wall. It is a constant reminder of hope, faith, innocence, and the miracle of the healing brain.

CHAPTER 8

How Do I Take Care of My Son?

It's 8 a.m. and the alarm clock has gone off twice already. Candy feels overwhelmingly exhausted, and she is experiencing intense pain and aching throughout her entire body. The thought of getting out of bed seems like too much to bear. She spends 40 minutes trying to get herself up, so she can get her eight-year-old son ready for school.

"Wake up honey," she says to her son with a fake smile, trying to hide the pain and discomfort she is in. She spends the next 45 minutes just managing to get him dressed and feed him a bowl of cereal. Secretly, she is counting down the minutes until she can go back to bed again.

When Candy finally gets her son off to school, she comes back home, goes immediately back to bed, and sets her alarm clock in time to cheerlead herself out of bed again in the afternoon when its time to pick up her son from school. On a good day, she might be able to stay up for 30 to 45 minutes. Most often, however, she has to go lie down for three to four hours at a time before she could even contemplate doing anything. Life was down to the absolute basics, and some days, even that was a stretch.

She safeguards her energy like a precious commodity, as she knows that there is always a cost analysis associated with any task. If she goes to the store, she knows that she will spend the next three hours in bed trying to recover. Sleep is the only thing that her body wants, just sleep. Yet no matter how much sleep she gets, she continues to feel exhausted all of the time. She is in a constant state of brain fog, with little ability to focus on anything. The pain and exhaustion is almost more than she can take. She feels as if she is slowly dying. Life has become a matter of survival, just trying to make it through the next minute, the next hour, the next day.

And on top of the chronic exhaustion, she has also developed a super-human sense of smell and can pick up on any chemicals in the environment. Perfumes and fabric softener fumes have become the number one enemy, and any exposure causes additional neurological symptoms along with a complete energy crash. Going for a walk is now even more challenging than it was before, not only because of the chronic fatigue and pain, but also because she has to worry about the next sudden 'dryer attack'.

On her worst days, Candy couldn't function at all. She would lay in bed, unable to get up, and she had to call on others to come and take care of her and her son. On these days, she was unable to take care of her own basic needs.

When Candy realized that something was really wrong, she went to see her doctor. On top of exhaustion, she was also experiencing a lot of abdominal and back pain. Her doctor simply told her, "Oh, you're just stressed," and suggested that she go home and rest. As you can imagine, this was not helpful at all. It took about six months to get a diagnosis of chronic fatigue syndrome (CFS). However, labeling her illness was not much help because, even with the diagnosis, there was nothing that the conventional medical system could do for her.

With little to no help from the mainstream medical system, Candy explored all avenues of healing. She tried Chinese medicine, which did manage to help with some of the pain, but it didn't help with the fatigue. She also did acupuncture and went to a naturopathic doctor. She tried vitamin C boosts and also tried chelation to remove heavy metals. In fact, Candy had several sessions of chelation, but she could not tolerate this treatment very well. It was too much for her body, given the fragile state that she was already in. She also tried different forms of counseling, thinking that maybe it was some kind of psychological or emotional issue that she could resolve. As a counselor herself, Candy was well informed about the subtleties and complexities of illness. She was willing to explore the possibility that perhaps it was an emotional issue or a mental health issue. However, counseling also proved not to be helpful.

Candy describes this time in her life:

> *On my really bad days I would wake up in the morning so achy and tired that I literally could not move. And it would take me anywhere from 20 minutes to 40 minutes to cheerlead myself enough to physically get out of bed. And on those days, I wasn't able to take my son to school, so either I would have to find somebody to drive him to school, or he would end up having to stay home with me. I would be lucky if I was able to get him and myself a bowl of cereal before having to go back to bed. And I would be in bed all day and sleep as long as I could possibly sleep.*
>
> *So basically, my life as I knew it was shut down. I had no outside extracurricular activities, I couldn't do work. I could barely look after myself, let alone my child, and so my life just became about survival, about doing the very basics, making sure that, you know, we had food, and the house was somewhat clean, and that was about it. And the multiple chemical sensitivities, I had to be very care-*

ful about where I went and who I was around. If I ran into somebody wearing perfume even in passing, I would instantly develop a really bad headache, and I would have to physically remove myself and often go lie down for a couple of hours before it would pass to the point where I was functioning again. While walking the dog if I smelled fabric softener from a neighbourhood laundry vent, it would be enough to induce a headache and nausea, and I would have to instantly remove myself. So that also limited me in what I was able to do and where I was able to go, and whom I was able to be around.

This whole experience was really difficult emotionally. I lost so much faith in life, in how I was going to move forward. My brain was so foggy and unclear that it was even difficult for me at times to process what was really going on, and hard, some days, not to be in tears all day, not knowing, whether tomorrow was going to be better or worse.

It was really difficult for me to be there for my son physically, let alone mentally and emotionally. We were having a conversation the other day, actually, and it came out that he was really worried. At one point, he thought I was going to die. And so did I, to be honest with you. That wasn't something that I had shared with him. But it affected his level of anxiety; it affected his ability to perform in school. It affected his ability to be away from me because he was worried about me, and so, of course that added to my stress levels and my ability to function because I had this little person glued to my side wondering what was going to happen.

There were times when I thought I was literally dying. I was a single parent without support, and I didn't know what to do. I didn't have any help. At one point, I even contemplated giving up custody of my son because I didn't *know how I could care for him. I wondered if he might be better off with my sister who lives in Bermuda. You can imagine that I would rarely see him if that happened. It's still very heartbreaking to think about, even to this day.*

Candy heard about the Dynamic Neural Retraining System™ through a friend. Her friend had read an article that I wrote for the Kelowna Capital News and had sent Candy an email suggesting that she might be interested in the program. Candy checked out the website and looked at some of the testimonials. Her first thought, as it is with a lot of people, was that the program seemed too good to be true. However, Candy saw the program as an opportunity to explore something different. She had tried so many different therapies already, and she had nothing to lose, and potentially everything to gain. And she thought that, if the program was half as good as the people on the website were claiming, then this could make a huge difference in her life.

Candy signed up for a program that I taught in Victoria in 2009.

Candy describes how the DNRS program was different than anything else that she has tried:

Well, first of all, Annie really made the program accessible to everyone in her awareness of the needs of the group and being environmentally aware. She ensured that no one was wearing any scented products so that the environment was good for everyone. Also, her passion about her work definitely comes across when she's facilitating. And her authenticity and her realness about her own experience makes it easy to connect with her on that level and to understand that this is a real person up here, sharing something that has worked for her. And that makes it so much more valuable, and so much more real, to be able to take a training system from someone who understands where you're at, and can relate to what you're going through, and can provide that guidance and a pathway out.

Through the program, I learned the tools that I needed to heal myself, so I could go away and do it myself. Which was a big factor, as opposed to coming back for regular treatments or having somebody try and do something to me. It was me helping to reorganize my own brain.

The program is also different in the sense that I learned that it was a brain injury that was creating the symptoms that I was experiencing. This was important for a few reasons. One of them being that it wasn't my fault – I didn't create this issue. Or the other part, which I think tends to be a prevalent mentality out there, is that it's all in my head because there wasn't something that showed up in the blood tests or the medical exams that I did. The program really helped me to understand that this isn't something in my mind or something that I'm just creating, or that I can make it go away by thinking positively or doing something different in that regard. The program really gave me the practical tools to go ahead and retrain my brain, to understand what was going on first of all, and then to retrain my brain so that my symptoms could decrease, and I could get on with my life.

By far, the hardest part about having a limbic system impairment was that it affected Candy's ability to parent. As a single mother, this was clearly a great concern, and Candy knew that the illness was also affecting her son in a big way. Recovering from limbic system impairment meant that Candy could get back to a normal everyday life and finally be the parent that she wanted to be. Candy speaks to her ability to be there for her son and how this is different:

WIRED FOR HEALING

My ability to be there for him and to function as a normal parent and to do activities with him has increased. We have a great relationship, and we can spend quality time together. And I don't feel like I'm constantly disappointing him by saying, "Well, maybe, but we'll have to see how my energy is. Maybe I can take you swimming. Maybe we can go for a hike. We'll see." And then, disappointing him when Saturday rolls around, and I'm not functioning. That is probably one of the biggest positive factors in my life after having done the DNRS program, that I can be the kind of parent that I want to be, and that is so important. My son is a lot more independent and a lot more emotionally mature and stable than he was before.

When I asked Candy what she can do now that she couldn't do before, she replied:

I can do the simple basic things in life, like having a normal routine – knowing that I can get up in the morning, and I can function throughout the day. Having more time and energy to spend with my son, so doing after-school activities, making plans for the weekend and being able to know that I'll have the energy to support following through on those plans and being more physically active. Spending more time outdoors, not worrying about going to a restaurant or going to the movies. Being able to do those kinds of things that I wasn't able to do before, or would really have to carefully consider depending on how I was feeling, or have to change my plans at the last minute if my energy wasn't there to support that.

So I really feel like my life is getting back to the point where I have some sense of normalcy, that I can do things that the average person can do. Now I'm at the point where I have gone back to work part time, which is really exciting for me. I wasn't sure, prior to doing the program, that was even going to be a possibility. I'm currently working a couple half-days a week and looking at increasing that in the very near future. And that's exciting for me. It's giving me that sense of accomplishment and pride that I wasn't sure I was going to be able to attain again.

When Candy was asked about her thoughts on the link between the environment and limbic system dysfunction, she replied:

I definitely think there is a link between environmental factors and multiple chemical sensitivities for sure, and quite possibly other limbic system injuries. I think that our bodies can only handle so much of an assault, and when we're being assaulted from all directions with air pollution, water pollution, our food being genetically modified and chemically sprayed – that all has a huge impact on our health, our immune systems, and our ability to not only remain healthy, but to fight illnesses when they arise. So I see this as a huge factor. Even though I don't have multiple chemical sensitivities anymore, I choose to use natural cleaning products in my house still, I choose to use unscented laundry detergent because I know that it makes a difference. And I think if we look at the number of people who are struggling with environmental illnesses and how that's exponentially increasing, it's a sign that we need to change how we live in this world. I love that Annie created the program from a platform of environmental awareness, as she really understands this pivotal link. She is also promoting environmental awareness in the things that we can do to improve or promote that awareness and ways that we can tread lightly in our world, to improve how we treat our environment and things that we can do to make a difference.

When Candy was asked what she would say to someone else who is still suffering, she replied:

> *I would really encourage them to take this program. You know, what have you got to lose? It's made such a profound difference in my life. I've kept in touch with some of the peers that I went to the program with, and I've seen the profound difference that it's made for them as well. It's really worth the time and effort to go and to do this training and to empower yourself to retrain your brain and make a difference in your life. I would never have believed that a normal life would have been possible. And yet, here I am. So I would really encourage people to give it a try and to see for themselves. And for those who can't make it to the in-person program and are doing the DVD program from their home, I would strongly encourage you to stick to it and to practise, and to really put in the effort. You need to stick with it to retrain your brain to get your brain working in this new neural pathway. Some people see results right away, they get that instant shift. And then there are others who take a little bit longer to recognize those shifts, or the shifts are subtle, so they're not necessarily as obvious right away. But I think the important thing is to keep at it, to practise, practise, practise, an hour a day, every day, for six months. And to know that even if you're not one of those people who gets that instantaneous shift, that*

maybe sometimes it takes a little bit longer for our brains to come online and make those new neural connections. To know that it will, and to know that there are lots of people who don't get that instantaneous 'wow factor' result, but who are diligent in their practice and in following through, and in the long term, see the exact same results as those who maybe got that initial burst of something. So really, for those of you who might be feeling a little bit disheartened that you're not making that progress as quickly as you might like to, just stick with it, and give this a fair shot, because it will make a difference, and it's that practice component that ensures that it does make a difference over the long haul.

And also know that there are, as you're doing this, probably thousands of other people who are walking the same path that you're walking at this moment, and that you aren't alone in this process. There is support there for you and to really give it your all, because it's worth it, the results are worth it.

Give it a try, go in with an open mind, and you will be amazed with what you can accomplish. You don't have to suffer anymore.

When I first heard about the program, it sounded too good to be true, almost like a fairy tale. But the Dynamic Neural Retraining System has given me the opportunity to engage with life again. Before that, I was really in a position where it didn't even feel like living. I mean, I was in bed all day, barely surviving, in very much a survival mode, without a lot of excitement in my life, or hope in my life. And this program has really given me the opportunity to get back out there and engage with life. I can do the activities I want to do. I can be there with my son and *play with him and go out and socialize with people in the evenings without being exhausted and having to go back to bed, or worrying about if someone's wearing perfume or not. So it's really given me that opportunity to get my life back and to be excited about what the future might hold.*

To others who are suffering, I would say, absolutely, without question, give this a chance. It is a fairy tale where dreams do come true, and it's amazing!

Candy graduated from the program in 2009 and fully recovered from Chronic Fatigue Syndrome and Multiple Chemical Sensitivities through the DNRS program. In fact, she is such a firm believer in the healing power of neuroplasticity and was so inspired by her recovery that she wanted to join the DNRS team. Prior to taking the DNRS Program, Candy held a Masters degree in counseling psychology and was already a practicing Registered Clinical Counselor and a Canadian Certified Counselor that specialized in the areas of trauma and chronic pain. In 2010, Candy became a certified Dynamic Neural Retraining System™ facilitator. She is also a senior DNRS Coach and Coaching Instructor.

CHAPTER 9

The Hazards of Living the American Dream

In 2001, Kevin was living the American dream. He was happily married, had three beautiful children and he had a job that he loved. He was living in Minneapolis, Minnesota, working for a high-tech company and making a lot of money. There was a lot of stress involved with his job, but he didn't mind it that much; in fact, it kind of made him tick. Life was going so well that Kevin and his wife Christy decided that it was time to purchase their dream home. Kevin refers to this home as the McMansion.

Unfortunately, what Kevin and Christy did not realize was that their new dream was about to turn into their worst nightmare. There was mould in the house. This can be very difficult to detect, and often isn't – until it's too late. Within a week of moving in, Christy started developing symptoms of fibromyalgia. Kevin's symptoms of environmental illness were slower to develop; however, his health, too, began to deteriorate. Kevin told me:

> I would get 'spots' – like an infection where my tonsils used to be. For a week at a time, I would have cold, or flu-like symptoms, congestion, and sore throat. I had my tonsils out when I was 30, so I thought that must be the problem. But the symptoms just kept getting worse.

Eventually Kevin had a biopsy of the throat spots, but the tests came back inconclusive. He was also cycling in and out of feeling like he had the flu for weeks at a time, and then feel fine. He also started to become sensitive to fragrances and to the chemicals found in personal hygiene products, cleaning products, and perfumes.

Gradually his life became consumed by illness, however Kevin was diligent in his quest to find healing. But the symptoms continued to worsen, and often Kevin felt as if he was being poisoned and was dying a slow, torturous death. His body was reacting to more and more stimuli, and with every episode, the symptoms became more severe. He went to visit an endless list of doctors, allergists, and every kind of specialist imaginable to find answers and solutions to his ailing health. Unfortunately, time and time again, he felt disappointed and discouraged when the 'treatment of the month' did not work and his condition continued to get worse. Finally, he went to the Mayo Clinic. He was almost certain that he would find the answers to his ailing health there, as they had the top specialists working together as a team to figure it out. As Kevin recalls:

> They ran every test imaginable and the 'great' news was, when everything was all said and done, they came in and gave me a clean bill of health. They told me, "you are perfectly healthy." They went through this long list of heart, lung capacity, and every other test and claimed that I was healthy. Even though the reality was that I was sick all the time.

Kevin's symptoms were very real, and extremely disabling, yet they could not be measured. How could that be? Like many people who are suffering from limbic system-related illnesses, Kevin felt increasingly hopeless and very discouraged. The lack of validation from the medical community and the isolation was an added burden. So back home he went. As the symptoms continued to get worse, Kevin was finding it more and more difficult to function in the world. Things like strong odours would make Kevin's eyes go bright red. He couldn't go to the mailbox because there were pesticides or herbicides in the yard. He couldn't be outside if anyone on his street was doing their laundry due to chemicals from the dryer exhaust.

Understandably, this also affected his ability to work. The list of new things that he was reacting to was growing larger and larger by the day. Any kind of exposure to chemicals or mould was now causing physical, cognitive, and emotional symptoms. Sadly, the only option was to move out of the house as it was making him too sick. At the time, they still had their old home, and Kevin moved back there. But by this time, he had also become sensitive to stimuli in his old house where he had lived for years without any problems. Kevin says:

> I kept getting sicker, and eventually I couldn't live in the new house. We still had the other house, and I was able to stay in two of the bedrooms there. However, I couldn't go in the kitchen or downstairs. I had to reduce my exposure to any kinds of chemicals. I was unable to think, feel, or remember – so I was unable to go to work. I couldn't go into buildings. I worked in those two rooms at home. Even at home, I couldn't work for more than two hours at a time.

In 2009, knowing that he had to take matters into his own hands, Kevin came up with an elaborate and courageous plan to find the best possible place to live. Eventually, he found that warm and dry climates seemed to be the best.

In a desperate attempt to recover, Kevin and his wife bought a small piece of land in New Mexico. They retrofitted a trailer with non-toxic materials and Kevin moved on to their remote property. He decided to go there alone, thinking that perhaps this place would help him recover and then he could move back with his family some day. As he describes this time:

> One of my lowest points was when I realized there was only one way to make a change – I had to get out. In December of 2009, I started living in my older model, off-gassed minivan. I got in the van and took off. I took myself all over the country to see if I felt better or worse in different situations. I kept a log of how I felt in different places and what triggered me. Like how my eyes looked, how my digestion was, etc. I kept this log while driving across the country.
>
> I found that warmer, dryer places seemed to be better. Eventually, we bought a small lot on the mesa and that's when we got the trailer. I moved there by myself to try and recover. Once I got there my life got really small.
>
> I had to leave my family and live by myself in the trailer. I had no visitors, and I had to have other people shop for me. I was alone and living in the middle of nowhere. Multiple chemical sensitivity symptoms made my life very small, constrained, and narrow.
>
> When my family did come to visit me, they would have to put all of their clothes in a bag and take a shower using my personal hygiene products and then wear clothes that I had for them. It was like being in jail, and they came to visit me in my cell.

Although living in the trailer and having great outdoor air quality was better for Kevin, his symptoms were not diminishing. By now, Kevin was suffering from extreme cognitive impairment and what he describes as severe brain fog. Life was going at a snail's pace, and he was only capable of performing very basic tasks. In his words:

> Going to the grocery store was really tough. I used a shopping list to keep track of things that I needed to buy but could not keep focused on the list due to the brain fog and confusion from the exposure to chemicals in the grocery store. I had a hard time just reading the list. I would walk around aimlessly wondering if I had already picked up that item or not. I would accidently lock my keys in the car. My memory was so bad that I could not make a simple meal like oatmeal. I could not keep track of how many cups of water I had put into the pot. I could not count to three, I would lose track. I would have to put one finger on the countertop at a time to indicate how many cups I had already poured. Even then I would lose track. I would do it over and over again. It was terrifying not being able to do something that simple. My ability to remember was gone.

Kevin also realized that his emotional state had changed dramatically. Understandably, he was feeling depressed because of his dire situation. But it was more than that. He felt disconnected emotionally to most everything:

> Over the course of those six to seven years, there was no joy. I was depressed. I had no feelings of affection – there simply just wasn't anything there. My memory was gone. My libido was completely gone. I had a general lack of feeling and didn't feel bad about doing something bad. I had no moral compass. I was really judgmental and negative in general. The one emotion that was left, for whatever

reason, was anger. Specific exposures to chemicals would immediately trigger bursts of anger.

Kevin continued to look for answers to his strange illness, and he started to see an environmental doctor in Santa Fe, New Mexico. Although the doctor's treatments had worked to decrease chemical sensitivities in other patients, the treatments were not working for Kevin. The doctor recommended that Kevin might want to try the DNRS, as some of his other patients had had some luck with it. According to Kevin:

> *When I heard about the program, I went to the website and looked at the testimonials, but I was skeptical. I had tried so many things and went to so many specialists, and none of them had worked. I just kept getting sicker. But I just had to give it a shot and see what happens. I thought it would be worth it to try something new. I signed up for the very next workshop up in Victoria, Canada, and I drove 1,600 miles one way to get there.*

Although Kevin was clearly not well during the program, I did start to notice some psychological and emotional changes in his behaviour. Kevin, however, did not become aware of them or acknowledge them until much later. In fact, he did not seem very hopeful at all when he left for his long journey back home. He seemed so discouraged that at one point during the program, he said that if he would have known what was involved in the program prior to attending that he would not have come. When the program finished, he quickly left and his parting words were: "If this actually works, that would be great." Those words were said with absolutely no emotion, and certainly no conviction.

In the following statement, Kevin's account of his trip to

Victoria is a clear depiction of how entrenched his brain was and how his limbic system disorder was affecting his perspective and emotional outlook on life. His focus was entirely on what was *not* working, noticing only the negative, and he was clearly very judgmental of others. He later told me:

> *The trip to the program was miserable. The weather was awful, I felt lousy, and there was construction everywhere. People were stupid.*

Kevin was courageous, though. Even though he was obviously struggling within the environment of the DNRS class, he stayed until the very end. He took lots of notes and participated; however, he was not very happy about it:

> *I was having a tough time in Victoria. I felt like I didn't make any progress. During the program I was really sick. I took lots of notes. I did the practice and the other things that were expected of me, but it was more mechanical and it didn't really connect.*

Part of the benefit of attending a live program is meeting other people who suffer from the same conditions. Kevin was particularly impressed by one of his classmates who is a highly educated, articulate and self-aware PhD. He recounts:

> *One of the turning points for me during the program was through one of my classmates, a highly educated PhD guy. I identified strongly with his intellect, and I watched him realize that this part of himself was preventing him from embracing the program. He wasn't allowing himself to fully participate. He wasn't allowing that part of his*

brain to do the work that he had to do. I identified with that very strongly because my skepticism was getting in my way, too. I realized that to get better, I had to work on all parts of me and let go of some of the beliefs I held before.

This was a big turning point for Kevin and gave him the opportunity to really embrace the fundamental idea of the program – that the brain was altered through trauma (mould, chemical, psychological stress) which in turn, altered its protective circuits. Afterwards, when we asked Kevin what he thought was different about the program, he replied:

What struck me as different was the idea that it was a brain injury. And I asked myself, "What if I had the cause and effect upside down? What if it wasn't just the exposure to chemicals that was causing the brain fog and the symptoms? What if the brain injury was making me more sensitive to chemicals?"

This new idea created an opening for Kevin to move forward and embrace the program, even though at that time he really didn't know if it would work at all. As an instructor, I could tell that he was already experiencing a shift in psychological and emotional states, but Kevin did not think that any changes took place during the program. This only became evident to him when he started his long journey back home. It was the first sign that the program was working for him.

Kevin states:

On the drive back, the same 1600-mile route, it seemed like everything was different. That was my clue that some-

thing had changed. Everyone had spent so much time making things nice, the road construction was making us safer, and the scenery was nicer. People looked better and smarter. The only thing that had changed was me, but I wasn't aware of it yet.

When Kevin returned to his retrofitted trailer, he was committed to practising the program. In the comfort of his trailer, he felt like he could really embrace the program and put into practice what he had learned. Within a week of returning home, he noticed that his symptoms were really starting to change:

> *I knew that the retraining was working shortly after I returned home. One of the concessions that my family made was to store their 'normal' clothes while visiting me. My wife would usually put their clothes in our storage trailer because there was something in the clothes that immediately triggered my symptoms. If I had to get something from the storage trailer, I would typically hold my breath, grab what I needed and quickly close the door to the trailer. About a week after I got back, I was looking for something in the storage trailer. I opened the trailer door and held my breath as usual, but I couldn't find what I was looking for. I eventually had to take another breath and then I realized I couldn't smell 'the toxic poison smell.' I stuck my face right in the clothes, took a big whiff, and I didn't have any reaction!*

As Kevin continued to improve, he was able to go to more and more places. His sense of freedom in the world was returning. When asked about a particular time in his recovery that really stood out for him as a big victory, Kevin recalled this amazing experience:

My wife and I were invited to go to town to see a musical performance that one of my coworkers was in. Now, because I was so much better, I felt like I could take this risk. We also decided to go for dinner beforehand because I was ready to try dining out again. I know it seems silly, but I chose the IHOP – because I like pancakes. Then we went to this musical theatre performance, and I was fine all the way through the performance! It was unbelievable! I met my coworker afterwards, and he was really surprised and happy to see me. On the way back to the car, I just started crying, and my wife thought something was wrong. I said to her, "I'm just so happy!" And she said, "If all it takes is IHOP and community theatre to make you happy, you might think about setting your sights a little higher."

From here, as Kevin continued to embrace his limbic system rehabilitation therapy, his symptoms continued to diminish. As a result, his life got bigger again, and he was able to engage in life in a normal way. He and his wife built an environmentally aware home on their land in New Mexico and that is where they live to this day. Remaining environmentally aware is just the smart thing to do. However, Kevin is no longer limited in where he can go and what he can do. Kevin remembers how things had changed after one hundred days into his retraining period:

Since the training, my life has gotten bigger again. I can think more clearly, I can work a full day. I can feel. I am happy again. I can go into buildings and see people. I can be part of the world again. I can move freely in the world, like most people take for granted.

I can feel positive emotions again – that mechanism is working again. All my hypersensitivities are turned down.

One of my concerns is that as I get better and do more and feel more, that I'll start to take life for granted and not appreciate the wonderful life I'm living. I'm genuinely happy and free again! I couldn't feel like this 100 days ago. My memory is back. Instead of an hour or two a day, I can work all day long. I can read a book and understand what's going on. I started a bucket list.

When Kevin volunteered to be a guest speaker at another program we were teaching, he got all choked up when he told the class that one of the items on his bucket list was to fly back to Minneapolis with his wife to visit their children for Christmas.

A year later when we interviewed Kevin again, he recounted the story to us and cried tears of joy when recalling that precious memory. He said:

My wife and I flew back to Minneapolis, to visit our kids for Christmas. It was the best trip of my life. My daughter recognized that things were better and used the line from the movie "Hook," when Peter Pan returns to Never-Never Land. In the movie, one of the lost boys doesn't recognize Peter as an adult until one day when he examines his face very closely, moving the skin on Robin William's face until he recognizes the little boy within. During our visit, my daughter lovingly grabbed my face one day and said, "So there you are Peter!"

I'm back. I can move through the world like this is my own planet now. I'm not an alien... I'm not allergic to everything on Earth. I'm going to hotels, flying on planes. I've got my life back. It's incredible.

When I asked Kevin what he would say to others who are still suffering, he replied:

> *Limbic system rehabilitation is just like climbing a mountain. You can't climb a mountain all at once. All you can do is work on the little patch of mountain right in front of you. Sometimes you make some progress, while other times all you can do is hunker down and wait for the storm to pass. Know that there are people above you with a rope in case you slip, and there are people below to catch you. Just keep focusing on that piece of mountain in front of you. From where I am now, the view is pretty spectacular.*

CHAPTER 10

From Wheelchair to Rollerblades

Lauren was 22 years old when she initially started to rewire her limbic system through the Dynamic Neural Retraining System DVDs. At that time, however, Lauren could not actually watch the DVDs on her television or computer due to extreme light and sound sensitivities. Minor sounds would startle her and activate a movement disorder with full-body twitching and shaking. In order for Lauren to just listen to the DVDs, her loving father had creatively stripped the sound track from the DVDs and slowed down the audio to a speed that Lauren could both tolerate and follow along with.

Before DNRS, Lauren's resting heart rate was twice its normal rate, as though she was constantly running in place, causing a lot of fatigue. It continued to worsen over time, until Lauren was unable to sit or stand for more than 2 minutes at a time. Due to the rapid heart rate, chest pain, blood pooling in her legs, and loss of consciousness, Lauren was mostly confined to lying in a reclining wheelchair or her bed. She barely had time to shower before her blood pressure plummeted. Lauren ate all her meals lying face down on a chaise lounge with her food served on a tray on the floor; at times, when her arm was too physically weak and sore to lift it to her mouth, her mother had to feed her.

The latest diagnosis in a string of illnesses was postural orthostatic tachycardia syndrome (POTS).

Although Lauren did make some progress listening to the DNRS DVDs, she still had a long way to go, and she was quickly giving up hope that recovery was even possible. I fondly remember interviewing Lauren on the phone to see if she would be a good candidate for the in-person program. She was frustrated with being ill and really seemed to be at a crossroads in her journey. Through tears, Lauren described her frustration to me. She thought that it was time to deal with the reality of living life as a person with a disability, rather than having hope that her life could be any different. It just seemed like having hope was counterproductive and so disappointing when time and time again, the various treatments that she underwent did not work. I really understood how Lauren could feel that way, especially given the fact that she had been to 35 specialists, and she had been sick since the age of 12. She just wanted to come to a place of acceptance of her disabilities and felt that her parents needed to come to this realization as well.

While I agree in principle that we need to come to a place of acceptance with life, this is not a position that I take when dealing with limbic system-related illnesses. I explained to Lauren that although she had been to see numerous specialists, they had not explored how a maladapted stress response could influence the numerous illnesses that she had been diagnosed with. I then went on to remind her of the subtle but positive changes that she was already experiencing with the DVDs and reassured her that attending the in-person program would be a positive experience for her.

She agreed that the in-person program was a good idea, but unbeknownst to me, she was thinking that the program would not work for her. And who can really blame her? If 35 different specialists and countless alternative practitioners could not help her, how could I? After all, I do not have a medical degree, and I am not a doctor. Lauren agreed to attend the in-person program strictly because she was grateful for the opportunity to leave her four walls for a few days. She really did not believe that this would be the catalyst to her recovery.

I remember the first time I saw Lauren at the Santa Fe program in 2011. Honestly, the first thing that I noticed was that she was in a reclining wheelchair and how out of place this seemed for such a beautiful, young woman. At 22 years of age, Lauren was basically living most of her life either in bed or in a reclining wheelchair. She had a very soft-spoken voice and greeted me with a big smile. I also noticed that her voice was weak and her breathing was laboured. Her mother, Cheri, was basically Lauren's caretaker, accompanied her. Cheri did not attend the program but was there to help care for and support Lauren.

The group dynamic inspired Lauren, and over the next 5 days, she applied herself completely to the program. Her enthusiasm and dedication were absolutely infectious. As it turns out, attending the in-person program gave Lauren the complete understanding that she needed to implement the program in the best possible way. She possessed the motivation and dedication to practice the DNRS program with the conviction of an Olympic athlete. Day by day, she freed herself from the physical prison of illness that had once held her captive for so long.

In order to really understand how liberating Lauren's recovery was, it might be best to hear about her history from her mother Cheri, who meticulously documented Lauren's journey of illness and recovery. Lauren's health issues started when she was only twelve years old. Below is a loving parent's perspective of illness and a summary of the health concerns and treatments that Lauren underwent prior to the Dynamic Neural Retraining System™ Program:

For those parents with chronically ill children, struggling to cope with their poorly understood conditions, I offer our own story as a beacon of hope to you. I pray that our experiences will direct you to the most effective treatments for your situation, with a minimum of financial and emotional burden.

A little about our family: I am a retired medical technologist/ microbiologist and my husband is a computer engineer/manager. We have two beautiful daughters, and for many years, we were all healthy and happy. Life was good. While my husband and I both have sensitive natures, and our children especially so, this reflects the genetic component of what was to come into our lives. At this time, we were not aware of the fearfulness our younger daughter Lauren carried within her from a very young age, nor can we think of any plausible explanation for this feeling other than she was simply 'wired' this way. While her general behavior seemed perfectly normal, as a toddler, she often found it overly stimulating to hold hands with others. What I thought was simply a quirk foreshadowed something more telling. When Lauren was eight, she fell ill with a serious viral infection that demyelinated nerve fibers in parts of her legs; she could not bear weight on them for four months before she spontaneously recovered. Many doctors have speculated that this event further altered her nervous system and manifested years later after other triggers arose.

Growing up, Lauren's personality was highly determined, academic, and athletic. While she could be very social and charming, her rule-oriented, 'glass half empty' thinking patterns took a toll by her high school years. At this time, other significant stressors came into play, especially her older sister's difficult battle with chronic pain *and anxiety from Lyme disease, contracted during a visit with family and friends back east. Here is Lauren's journey, in a nutshell:*

PROGRESSION OF SYMPTOMS AND DIAGNOSES:

Spring 2002: Lauren's first obvious symptom was exercise-induced asthma when running, which began at age twelve. Her likely trigger was stress when we moved suddenly from New Jersey to Colorado, leaving behind many close friends and the abundance of trees and wildlife she adored there.

Spring 2005: Developed pollen allergies and painful menstrual cycles.

Spring 2006: Explosion of allergies; skin tests positive to 54 of 76 antigens (pollen and shellfish). Allergy shots three times a week for two and a half years: therapeutic dose never reached due to hypersensitive immune response. Other symptoms consisted of year-round congestion and sinus infections, poor sleep, stomach pain, acid reflux and digestive issues.

Fall 2008: When starting college, she contracted multiple concurrent infections. Strep throat and sinusitis/bronchitis, both treated with antibiotics; Candida infection followed, treated with Diflucan. Food sensitivities increased. As a first-year engineering student, Lauren implemented a food elimination diet, eating only non-processed, organic, gluten/egg/dairy-free low carbohydrate foods, with grass-fed meats (her meals were made at home and brought to her dorm fridge). Lauren was self-conscious eating her "special" meals with others in the dining hall, so she ate alone in her dorm room. This caused more feelings of isolation and increased fear of the physical changes occurring in her body, which she tried harder than ever to suppress.

July 2009: Near fainting, pronounced fatigue, and stomach issues worsen. Stage III adrenal exhaustion and hypochlorhydria diagnosed.

November 2009: Mononucleosis infection causing tachycardia (resting heart rate 90-100), extreme fatigue, shortness of breath, nausea, joint pain, increased anxiety.

Spring 2010: Irritable bowel syndrome diagnosed by primary physician, verified by gastroenterologist. Psychiatrist noted sleep disorder and prescribed Seroquel which caused a chemical injury affecting dopamine receptors, resulting in a movement disorder triggered by any sensory overload.

Summer 2010: Two weeks after a lumbar puncture for a multiple sclerosis study, Lauren suffered prolonged nerve pain from the procedure. Resting heart rate jumped to 115. Sound and light sensitivity became more evident. Fibromyalgia and chronic fatigue syndrome (CFS) diagnosed by rheumatologist and CFS Specialist.

Fall/winter 2010: two visits to Mayo Clinic (Rochester, MN). Tachycardia due to postural orthostatic tachycardia syndrome (POTS), and pollen/food allergy syndrome diagnosed. Previous diagnoses of fibromyalgia, chronic fatigue syndrome, and irritable bowel syndrome also verified by Mayo. Began twelve-month treatment contract with a fibromyalgia & fatigue center in Denver, founded by a renowned MD specialist.

Spring/Summer 2011: Multiple bacterial urinary tract infections and Candida infections after viral treatment with Valcyte (begun 1/3/11) for elevated Epstein-Barr and HHV-6 titers. Symptoms also included extreme fatigue, weight loss, diarrhea, bruising/bleeding, and extensive hair loss. Narcolepsy diagnosed in March following abnormal multiple sleep latency test.

Fall 2011: Constant chest pain began, causing further disability requiring full-time assistance. Lauren moved from her apartment in Boulder to home. Candida infection flourished and she was prescribed daily oral Diflucan for 12 consecutive weeks, along with other anti-yeast treatments.

Jan 2012: Functional medicine specialist diagnosed mitochondrial dysfunction due to high oxidative stress on bioimpedance analysis test, (her cell function was on the level of an elderly woman), and suspected additional latent infections (Babesia, Bartonella, Borrelia).

Spring/Summer 2012: As mitochondrial dysfunction and immune system treatments were implemented, light and sound sensitivity became severe, with intolerance of benign noises (stuffed cotton in ears to muffle sound) and inability to view computer screens or TV due to instant migraine symptoms. Reflections and small patches of sunlight were painful as well. Chest pain also worsened and Lauren could *no longer sit upright; was able to stand for only two to three minutes at a time before blood pooling in legs (acral cyanosis) caused low blood pressure and compensative tachycardia. Discontinuation of all newer treatments did not resolve nervous system hypersensitivity. Weight dropped to 98 lbs. despite eating five to six full MD-approved meals/day. Organic grass-fed bison bone broth to heal intestines and improve adrenal function helped to restore some weight. Anxiety and depression worsened, and daily episodes of rage and thoughts of suicide continued. Lauren required continual assistance. Gerry & I hired a nursing student, Amanda, to help twice a week with her full time care, and together we worked as a team. Lauren's nervous system, immune system, endocrine system, and digestive system were compromised. While we tried our best to remain upbeat in front of Lauren, inside we were terrified. While her doctors tried to make educated guesses on how to proceed, they really did not know how to directly address this scenario and had never experienced such a case. It is difficult for me to fully convey just how desperate and frightening Lauren's situation was; she was caught in a downward spiral and we feared she would not survive if this trend did not reverse soon. Feelings of anxiety, rage and depression were at a peak. Lauren was so uncomfortable, both physically and emotionally in every waking moment that she wanted to die just to end the suffering.*

Fall 2012: Holistic psychiatrist seen to help balance neurotransmitters; carefully reduced/changed many medications/supplements. Tilt-in-Space wheelchair ordered. We were introduced to the DNRS Program by her functional medicine MD. While we were a little unsure at first that brain retraining could help Lauren's situation, we figured it would cause no harm, and we didn't want to leave any stone unturned. Lauren listened to the program after her Dad copied the audio track onto CDs (using her specialized player that slows down speech without altering the pitch since she could not process words at a normal speed). While she had some success with light and sound tolerance, within two weeks, she hit 'roadblocks' and became discouraged.

Winter 2013: Since Lauren was so physically and emotionally overwhelmed at this time, she developed resistance to the retraining. One of her limbic system loops was fear of failure, but another was a fear of success (and the many changes that would bring), leading to 'mental gridlock,' even though it was clear that the brain retraining was responsible for her improvements.

Spring 2013: When we received the announcement of the upcoming DNRS seminars, I was not hopeful that Lauren would be open to attending because of her 'limbic system loop' regarding brain retraining. It was a personal story of someone else's recovery (very similar to her own) included in a newsletter from Annie Hopper that helped her to consider the idea. Initially she agreed to go because traveling anywhere would feel like a vacation. Lauren was the first to admit that she was very resistant to attending the seminar since she wasn't fully convinced this process could really solve all her issues, particularly since she had so many conditions and her symptoms were so severe.

She later told me that she had no plans to restart the practice, but after meeting the other people at the seminar, with the supportive group dynamic, it was infectious! The seminar allows for more in-depth explanations with suggestions for customizing one's practice, and Lauren quickly made the necessary remaining connections in her understanding of the program.

Each day, even during the seminar itself, she had a slew of new successes: improved sleep, more energy, and a more positive outlook. In less than one month after the seminar, by consistently doing her retraining practice and appropriately challenging herself, Lauren learned to rollerblade (backwards too!), went bike riding, gardened and did yard work (with heat tolerance much improved), she attended a Rockies baseball game, can watch TV with us again, has been to movie theaters, and can now sit or stand for hours at a time! Even though it was still a physical challenge for her to perform these tasks, progress was clearly evident. She accomplished all these things without the use of her wheelchair, and it hasn't been used since.

Lauren also began to introduce new foods back into her diet: sometimes it went well and sometimes not, but as she persevered in her practice to control her limbic system stress response, her intestinal lining continued to heal and her immune system rebalanced. Within three months she could eat absolutely anything, even shellfish (which is usually considered to be a permanent allergy), with no adverse effects! So for the first time in years, Lauren was able to go out on "real dates" with her boyfriend Kevin (now husband), sit up in a chair and eat restaurant prepared food. In August, they traveled together to California to visit family and spent time at Disneyland and California Adventure, walked for hours, went on roller coasters and watched laser shows! In just over 4 month's time, Lauren's recovery was already nearly complete.

LAUREN'S TREATMENT HISTORY

Specialists: Since 2006, Lauren has seen a total of 35 medical doctors, including 6 at Mayo:

- CFS/fibromyalgia specialist (1)
- functional medicine MD (1)
- holistic MD (2)
- neurologist (3), autonomic specialist (1)
- cardiologist (2), electrophysiologist (4)
- rheumatologist (1)
- gastroenterologist (1)
- internal medicine MD (1)
- allergist/immunologist (4)
- ear, nose and throat specialist (ENT) (2)
- gynecologist (2)
- primary care MD (2)
- emergency room (ER) MDs (5)
- psychiatrist (2)
- sleep specialist (1)

TREATMENTS INCLUDED AN ARRAY OF PRESCRIPTION MEDICATIONS AND SUPPLEMENTS:

- beta blocker, various steroids, antibiotics, antifungals, antivirals, antidepressants, sleep aids, etc.
- nutritional and CFS supplements (>100 products)
- major auto-hemotherapy with ozone & UV light
- frequency specific microcurrent

Complementary treatments included dietary changes with avoidance of reactive foods, grain-free diet with grass-fed meats and organic produce, bison bone broth, high salt & fluid intake, thigh-high 30-40 Hg compression stockings, acupuncture (Chinese & Japanese), hypnotherapy, psychotherapy, chiropractic, biofeedback, neurofeedback, massage therapy, aromatherapy, healing sounds, guided meditation/mindfulness CDs, Reiki, NeuroEmotional Technique, Matrix Energetics and several other forms of energy healing/balancing, as well as spiritual/religious prayer/meditation.

In the past seven years, we have spent more than $100,000 in out-of-pocket expenses for Lauren's medical testing, treatments, and care. While our health insurance covered most of the 'conventional' costs, CFS supplements are not covered and coverage for alternative care such as chiropractic and acupuncture was very limited. The CFS doctors were all out-of-plan, which greatly reduced coverage.

While we were fortunate that our family had the financial resources to explore all avenues available to us, many of the recommended approaches we took made the situation worse. While a few of these treatments were mildly helpful, most were neutral, and some were quite harmful, causing additional infections or further nervous system stimulation/damage. Although the doctors we worked with were all experienced and well-meaning, we discovered that directly attacking latent infections or modulating the immune system caused excessive stimulation of the sympathetic nervous system, in turn adding to limbic system stimulation. Many of the 'energizing' CFS nutrients/supplements further contributed to nervous system hypersensitivity as well. In our experience, treating these secondary effects, while often supportive and necessary, did not lead to full recovery until the abnormal stress response was also controlled.

In recent years, neuroplastic techniques have been successfully developed for stroke and traumatic brain injury victims; DNRS applies neuroplastic techniques for those with limbic system dysfunction. This is the root cause of conditions such as MCS, Fibro, CFS, Post-Traumatic Stress Disorder, etc.; these diagnoses are simply the manifestations of the ways the brain becomes miswired due to physical/emotional trauma, prolonged stress, and/or infections. Very few doctors, even those trained in holistic or functional medicine, are aware of this 'top-down' relationship or that an intervention exists.

Of the myriad of treatments Lauren has trialed, the one that changed everything has been the neural retraining with the DNRS Program. When Lauren began the DVD program in early October, her condition was grim. While her limbic system was too impaired at that time to fully grasp the mindset and techniques, simply understanding the relationship of the limbic system to the chronic stimulation of her 'fight-or-flight' response was extremely helpful in explaining what this was doing in her body. With that knowledge, Lauren was able to make enough progress over the next few months such that attending the five day in-person session in April was physically possible. Meeting in person with Annie and Candy, the guest speakers, and fellow clients was extremely powerful for Lauren and made all the difference for her. Her recovery has already been swift and nothing short of a miracle!

Additionally, the information and tools in the DNRS program are applicable to everyone, not just those with chronic illness. Don't discount this program because it seems too simplistic—it is deceptively powerful!

Added to this is Lauren's powerful personal account of her recovery process. Needless to say, Lauren is very excited to share her story so that she can now give others the hope and faith to keep going and have the courage to try 'one more thing.'

The following is Lauren's five month update:

> *Just five months ago, I returned from the Dynamic Neural Retraining System seminar. There's no other way to describe my experiences other than, "life before Dynamic Neural Retraining – and after!"*
>
> *Before my illnesses hit hard, I was an engineering student at the University of Colorado at Boulder. I used to dance down the aisles in the grocery store, lift weights, rock climb, and laugh a lot. After multiple bacterial and fungal infections, I also contracted mono and developed POTS (postural orthostatic tachycardia syndrome). After a series of unsuccessful treatments which worsened my condition, I became unable to sit up or stand longer than a couple minutes at a time before chest pain and blood pooling in my legs required me to lie down. And because my nervous system had become so sensitized, even normal everyday sounds hurt my ears and would startle me. I was unable to look at a TV, computer, or cell phone screen without getting an instant migraine. I would try wearing sunglasses, but the weight of the glasses on my nose and ears were too painful. I also developed more and more sensitivities to foods, except for twelve things (and that included spices). My weight dropped to 98 lbs. even though I ate six or more meals a day. My parents even fed me at times because I was too weak to lift the food to my mouth. All I could do was lie in bed and listen to audiobooks on a special CD player*

that could slow the speed of speech so I wouldn't struggle to understand it. I had these symptoms for an entire year.

I now lift weights with Kevin, and I have more than doubled the weight I once benched, squatted, and dead-lifted when I began retraining four months ago. For years, we had dreamed of being able to work out together. It was an activity I truly enjoyed in high school and one that my power-lifter guy also appreciated. And taking dance classes again is such a gift!

What has been most fulfilling are all of the 'firsts' that Kevin and I have been able to experience five years after we met. Despite not knowing me while I was healthy (until now), he somehow always knew the person I was and who I could be. I am so grateful for his relentless faith in me. Being able to do what to some sounds trivial, for us, is a miracle. We've gone on our first date at a restaurant, and I actually ate the food made by the establishment (instead of bringing my own in Tupperware)! We have even gone on our first vacation – to Disneyland! It was an all-day, on-your-feet adventure where we ate everything, rode everything, and we just loved it! I've even gotten Kevin to take a salsa class with me! There are so many 'firsts' that now we pretty much expect them.

Looking back, I am so humbled by the memories I recall when my family had cared for me before my recovery. My mom became my best friend. She did everything with me and for me when I could not do it for myself. And my sister, when she did my make-up as I lay in bed, I remember her having the most gentle and loving touch. She made me feel so pretty. And when I was most doubtful, it was my dad that encouraged me. He knew the solution was out there and that we would find it. Because of his certainty, I believed it too.

Well, I wish I could say I was super into the Dynamic Neural Retraining System (DNRS) from the beginning, but that just wasn't the case. I was quite resistant to the idea that I had some say (any say actually) in my debilitating health conditions.

Here's how I would put it: you did nothing wrong to get to where you are healthwise (and feelings of frustration and despair towards the situation are completely understandable!), but your thoughts have the power to rewire faulty brain circuits that cause pain and suffering.

So back to my experience... at the very beginning, I couldn't commit to the six months of retraining practice like I was supposed to. First of all, I knew I couldn't wait that long to see improvement. Secondly, my situation was so severe I was sure that my recovery would take much longer than someone else with just mild or moderate symptoms. So the way things happened was that although I couldn't promise myself I would do this for six months, I gave it a real go for just that first day. It turned out that I had to remind myself of the program nearly every second. I was always catching myself and putting myself back on track. I began to see and feel improvement after just the first day. I continued to practice just because it made a discernible difference nearly every time I implemented the program. Most of the time, this just meant I felt a little calmer and more centered. It all improved in baby steps, but after the first night, I could reduce my sleep meds, sit up a couple moments longer than would usually be possible, and my sensitivity to fragrances greatly improved.

As far as thinking that I would take longer to heal because I'd been sick for so long and so severely, that couldn't have been further from what actually happened. It seemed like because I had so many symptoms, they began to melt away in multiples! For a few weeks, sometimes 6 symptoms improved in increments or even resolved every day. It was very exciting. After two months of retraining, I had gained so much momentum; it was like a game to see what would improve that day! The biggest change was that I could focus on the positive changes in my life, not the things I still wanted (and needed) to improve. You also learn how to measure your success differently; sometimes it was loading the dishwasher or putting on make-up that was the accomplishment! But it's all great and all deserving of a celebration.

What would Lauren say to others who are still suffering?

First of all, it is essential that you get the DVDs and/ or go to the seminar so you have a clear understanding of the program in its entirety. It's so important because a full understanding of how your brain works is crucial for applying the method. That way, you are sure of the concepts and process of retraining.

When someone has chronic pain or illness, the body is in 'fight-or-flight' mode to protect and communicate with the rest of the body that it's sick and in pain – that something's wrong. Overriding the overactive 'fight-or-flight' response allows your body to put its energy into healing and repairing.

There are many forms of trauma that affect brain function.

Viruses, bacteria, chemicals, emotional/psychological, and physical stress can cause brain trauma and catapult your brain into a 'fight-or-flight' state. This is measurable through the latest research in neuroscience. Also, your thoughts, feelings, behaviors, and life experiences are recorded in your brain through specific and well-worn neural circuits. Some of these unconscious neural circuits can actually be keeping your brain in a trauma cycle.

In the recovery process, it is vital to become aware of the patterns you are running, both conscious and unconscious, in order to change them. This takes insight, work, dedication, repetition, and a skill set that is best learned at the DNRS in-person seminar.

I was amazed at how I could actually be in charge of how my brain functions and how that transformed my state of health. In fact, everyone is amazed!! Even my doctors – many of whom did not understand the connection the limbic system has in regards to our overall health. The 35 specialists I had seen and my visits to the Mayo Clinic had been helpful in diagnosing many of my conditions, but determining how to recover was not well known. My suggested plan of action was to take medication to manage the symptoms and wait until I "grew out of it." However, Annie Hopper and the DNRS team could explain just what was happening, why it was happening, and how I could get better. I am so grateful I was able to attend the program to implement the training.

In time, the 'fight-or-flight' response no longer goes off inappropriately. When this response normalizes, your body's natural repair mechanisms resume. Through techniques in neuroplasticity, new and healthy brain connections develop while faulty connections are disconnected. That's when you feel better!

The symptoms of chronic pain are completely real. It is not just 'your imagination'. But you can retrain your *brain, and it's just like hitting the reset button. Recovering from chronic pain sounds like an uphill battle, but it's really much easier and more rewarding than you could ever imagine. Having the right tools make the impossible happen. So climb that mountain!!!*

LAUREN'S SIX MONTH UPDATE OCTOBER 23, 2013:

I met with my functional medicine doctor yesterday to document my improvement, and an orthostatic blood pressure test concluded that I no longer have postural orthostatic tachycardia syndrome (POTS)!

The test consists of comparing your heart rate and blood pressure when you're laying down for fifteen minutes and after standing for one minute. When I had POTS, my average resting heart rate was 135 bpm, and my blood pressure dropped to 80/60 upon standing (in addition to blacking out). THIS TIME, my resting heart rate was 75 bpm, and both my heart rate and blood pressure remained constant and didn't change after standing for the minute. In other words, I could not have passed more definitively. Very happy day!

Lauren goes on to say:

I look forward to applying all that I have learned from my brain retraining. Before my recovery, I knew it would feel amazing to be in good health once again, but what I'm experiencing is so much more remarkable than I could have imagined. I never thought my life could turn around so fast! My recovery is teaching me so many, invaluable lessons that will always serve me.

Many refer to my recovery as a miracle, but I think the real miracle is that my recovery occurred via the Dynamic Neural Retraining System, a method that can be taught to others so they can experience their own miracles. Improvement can come in waves or in incremental steps; the important thing is not to judge how it happens. I have faith in you – have faith in your recovery. It will be so humbling and a joy to look back on all that you've accomplished.

Thank you Lauren, for having the courage to try "one more thing." You are such a bright and shining spirit. You have the power to illuminate the entire world with your joy, enthusiasm, and love! Lauren has joined the DNRS team as a certified DNRS coach. Lauren and Kevin married in the summer of 2014. To learn more about Lauren, please visit her website at www.wheelchairtorollerblades.com.

When Food Becomes the Enemy

Judy weighed only 78 pounds when she attended the Dynamic Neural Retraining System™ program in November of 2012. At that time, Judy's eyes were hollow, her skin was grey, she was very weak, and in her own words, "looked like I just came out of a concentration camp."

Judy had suffered from severe food sensitivities for 17 years that she believes were exacerbated by various underlying conditions throughout her life, including hepatitis, candida, and Lyme disease. Judy went on to develop chronic fatigue syndrome, fibromyalgia, and chemical sensitivities.

As a registered nurse, Judy was educated and knowledgeable about the workings of the body. She did a lot of research on her own and had also been to countless medical professionals looking for answers. Judy and her husband had spent "in the hundreds of thousands of dollars" trying to find answers to her escalating health issues. Judy had tried elimination diets, candida diets, and rotation diets, yet nothing was working. No matter what she did, she was becoming more and more sensitive to food. As her sensitivities increased, she became unable to eat more than a handful of foods. Judy continued to lose weight, and her muscles were beginning to atrophy.

By December 2011, Judy's food sensitivities had become so

severe that she was barely able to eat anything. She could literally span her finger and thumb around her upper arm. Judy said, "I was losing foods by the day. I panicked. I could clearly see the writing on the wall and knew that if the illness continued to progress, it wouldn't be long before I would be unable to eat any foods."

Judy thinks that there were a number of different traumas in her life that contributed to the perfect storm that triggered limbic system dysfunction and a chronic maladapted stress response. Here's Judy's description of the series of events that led up to her limbic system trauma:

> I think this may have really started when I was born because my mom had severe post-partum depression and wasn't really able to really take care of me. Even then, my parents had a difficult time finding any baby food that I could tolerate. And then when I was 5 or 6, I had hepatitis B, and again, I was put on a special diet. It had to be a fat-free diet because that's how they treated it back then. I still remember that feeling of deprivation and how I really wanted those foods that I couldn't have. And then in my 30s, I was diagnosed with candida, and I went on a candida diet, and all that that entails. And then finally in my 40s, I got Lyme disease, which wasn't diagnosed right away.

By the time that Judy was diagnosed with Lyme disease in 2006, she was also suffering from chronic fatigue, fibromyalgia, chemical sensitivities and a rapidly expanding list of food sensitivities.

One thing that really stood out for Judy is that she could clearly see how limbic system dysfunction was operating with food sensitivities. She could understand that her brain was interpreting food in a distorted fashion and they were causing a change in psychological and emotional states. Judy clearly remembers a time when she had gone to a Thai food restaurant and she experienced a severe emotional and psychological reaction to foods that were previously okay until that day. On that particular day, she had eaten at that restaurant twice. Judy remembers the reaction as stepping into a dark abyss. She was experiencing paranoia along with sudden and severe depression. It took everything that she had to get through that night. From that point on, she had become fearful to eat the same foods as she did not know whether she could weather another reaction. Food had now become the enemy and eating was akin to playing Russian roulette. Judy became very vigilant about what she could eat and when. She tracked what her body was reacting to, what was okay, and what was not okay. This seemed to work until 2011 when the illness escalated again. Judy knew that she had to eat to stay alive, but her body and brain were reacting so violently to foods that she was unsure how she could survive.

By the end of 2011, she was losing foods by the day. Judy could only tolerate fish and a few leafy vegetables. She couldn't eat any oils, fat, or carbohydrates in any form. Her hormone levels were all over the place with low thyroid, sky-high cortisol, sky-high human growth hormone, and almost non-existent estrogen and progesterone. Her blood work prompted her doctors to test for a tumor. The tests the doctors wanted to perform involved radioactive dye, but Judy couldn't imagine how she might survive that when she couldn't even eat a pear! Confronting her doctors and declining the tests was yet another stress on her already overtaxed situation.

By this time, Judy was also suffering from extreme muscle wasting. She was extremely weak and found it incredibly challenging to even walk up a flight of stairs. She eventually had to apply for a parking sticker for people with disabilities because it was so hard to go to the grocery store and get the groceries back into the car. When her husband was away on business, they would have to hire someone to come in and do the dishes, as Judy was too weak to do them. She was shocked that her life had come to this.

Judy was living in survival mode all of the time with her entire focus on avoiding trigger foods and on trying to sustain life. Little did she know that things were about to get a lot worse before they got better. During this time frame, her loving husband, who was her main caretaker and support, suffered from a massive heart attack. Judy describes the moment that it happened:

> He was sitting on the couch and he hadn't been feeling good all day. I had gone out and then came back and asked how he was doing. He said that he was feeling much better and that was the last thing he said before he went down. I called 9-1-1, and they came, and they had to resuscitate him four times; three times at the house and once in the ambulance. And then he was in the hospital, in ICU on life support. So this was really the bottom for me. I'm a Registered Nurse, so I knew that I was the best person to be there with him. Not just because I'm his wife but because I know the system, and I know a little bit about what he was experiencing and suffering from. So I really wanted to be there for him, but I couldn't in the way that I wanted to. The whole thing was just so exhausting.

At this time Judy had already signed up to take the Dynamic Neural Retraining System™ program, but was unsure how she could leave her husband during this difficult time. Her husband was also her caretaker and was supposed to drive her to the program and be there to support her. Judy speaks about her determination to attend the program. Her husband had been released from the hospital for just over a week prior to the start date of the program.

> *I didn't know how I was going to do it. And yet I felt like 'I have to.' I just felt as if my life depended on it really. So we got a friend to come and stay with Barry, and then I had a friend come down with me and keep me company.*

Judy recognized after she started the DNRS program that the rest of the treatments that she tried were merely addressing the symptoms and not the root problem – the limbic system. She fully recognized that avoidance and the rotation diets were not working. During the five day program, using the tools that she was taught, her system started to shift, and she was slowly able to introduce more and more foods.

What followed over the six months after the DNRS program could be described as nothing less than remarkable.

What stands out about Judy's recovery story is that the physical changes are abundantly apparent. Of course, you cannot see limbic system dysfunction when looking at a person because a brain injury is invisible. However, in Judy's case, limbic system dysfunction was making it impossible for her to eat, so her illness was physically apparent, and she looked very emaciated. After attending the program and applying the tools to rewire her limbic system, Judy's physical appearance rapidly shifted. She was able to eat more foods and as a result was able to gain weight – sometimes at a pace of five pounds per week. Her friends and family were almost in a state of shock when they saw Judy just a couple of months after the program as she had gained over 20 pounds and was looking healthy and vibrant again.

Judy shares what her experience was like attending the program:

> For me, the program was fantastic because once I realized that I had these tools and that I could eat – I started eating! It all made sense that limbic system dysfunction was at the very root of the problem and that other treatments were merely addressing the symptoms, not the cause. It's like a hornet's nest, and you're trying to swat the individual hornets that come out of the nest instead of just dealing with the nest. This deals with the 'nest' – it goes to the root of the problem. When I realized what was happening, I had offered to Annie that I would take pictures of myself because I knew how bad I looked. I weighed myself as soon as I returned home because I knew that I was going to be gaining weight pretty quickly. That's when I found out that I only weighed 78 pounds. I looked like a holocaust victim.

After leaving the program, Judy felt empowered to take charge of her health. She describes this in the following:

> One thing that's been huge for me is recognizing that my limbic system's not in charge. Before the program, I didn't know that much about the limbic system. Even though I'm a registered nurse! We learned about the limbic system, but I never thought that it was my limbic system that was causing all of the problems. Before, as soon as I would get some kind of a reaction, some kind of a symptom, I just caved. I'd be avoiding foods, or whatever. So, realizing that I can control this has been such a relief for me. Because now I feel like I can manage my limbic system. So, that's been a real relief.

Judy immediately started gaining weight, her sensitivities decreased, her thyroid function normalized, her muscle strength and energy returned, and her skin colouring returned to normal again.

A defining moment when Judy knew that she was well on the road to recovery was the day she went to see a movie with her husband and some friends. Usually she would not have been able to go due to her various sensitivities. Just the smell of popcorn would give her a bad migraine, so until this time, going to movies was completely out of the question. Judy describes this victorious moment in time:

> In the past, chemical sensitivities kept me from going to the movies because the popcorn smell would give me horrible migraines. Just 2 months after I did the program, I went to the movies, and to my surprise, they had refurbished the movie theater. My initial feeling was just 'I should get out of here.' But we were with friends, and so I was embarrassed and I didn't want to leave. So I decided to practice my limbic system retraining exercises instead. And before I knew it, I was just watching the movie. I don't even remember at what point I stopped noticing the smells and was just watching the movie. It was such a success and I just felt so proud of myself.

Judy goes on to talk about all the things she can do now:

> Now I can go to restaurants, I can travel and stay at bed-and-breakfast hotels. I don't have to prepare and plan my meals ahead of time. If my system is stressed in any way, because the food issue is the weakest link, I can sense a slight increase in food sensitivities, but I don't worry about it. I

know what to do and I have the tools to deal with this. I can visit my daughter in her new apartment with new furniture. I can go where I want to. And I can fly on planes again. This is huge!! Before I attended the program, in January 2012, I flew to L.A., just a 2-hour flight, and my ankles looked like elephant legs, which I'm sure had something to do with the endocrine system. Just a few months ago, I flew again, and I wore the special socks. On the way there, nothing happened, so on the way back, I didn't even wear the special socks, and my ankles didn't swell. So, I can travel again. And I can walk up stairs! I went to a concert shortly after doing the program, maybe two months after doing the program, and the women's bathrooms were in the basement, and we were on the main level. The line-up for the bathroom was huge, and while waiting in line, this lady comes and says, "I can take you to another women's bathroom where there's no line." But that women's bathroom was on the top floor! So I had to go all the way up from the basement to the main floor, and then all the way up again to the top floor. And as I'm walking up the stairs, I realized, "I can do this, really, I can do this, this is awesome!!!"

Judy recognized that, for her, the program represented much more than a tool for recovery. She goes on to say:

I don't have a timeline about how long I will need to practice the program. In some ways I feel like I'm still learning more about the program and feel like this is something that I will do for the rest of my life. Because actually, the fact is, I really enjoy it! You know, I really enjoy doing it. It's so good for me – the joy that it's bringing me is significant. I'm just very grateful and appreciative!

After seeing the huge transformation in Judy, many of her friends and family have since taken the program. In fact, Judy's friend that drove her to the program has recovered from post-traumatic stress disorder using DNRS. Truly, rewiring the limbic system has a happiness ripple effect.

CHAPTER 12

High School Sucks

Tyffanee was thirteen years old when she started to develop multiple chemical sensitivities. According to Tyffanee, she doesn't really remember any single event that may have triggered the illness, although she does describe herself as fairly "anxious" in general. She worried a lot, big or small – things that she could control and those that she could not – she worried about them all. Even when thinking back to her childhood and her earliest memories of herself, she described herself as an Olympic worrier. Like all teenage girls, at age thirteen she was also going through some big hormonal shifts. Her family had just moved, and her parents had purchased a restaurant where she worked part time. Undoubtedly, there were new textiles off-gassing and renovations associated with this move that most likely contributed to the general load on her central nervous system.

Being a young teenager with chemical sensitivities comes with a unique set of challenges. Being different and being unable to socialize is very difficult when all you want to do is fit in with your peers. It was also proving to be more and more difficult for Tyffanee to attend regular public school due to the daily exposures that she would encounter. She changed schools a number of times, was sent to private school, and was finally homeschooled due to the severity of her sensitivities and reactions to any fragrant products or chemicals. Tyffanee wanted to go to school, and she wanted to have friends, but that was almost impossible as chemicals and fragrances are in the majority of personal hygiene products. As time went on, the illness progressed and so did the severity of her symptoms. All she wanted was to be a "normal kid". But she wasn't. Tyffanee remembers:

> When I first started getting sensitive, it wasn't too bad, but it progressed over the years to the point where I had to have my EpiPen with me, everywhere I went. School was really hard. I ended up graduating, but just barely. My parents had to bounce me around from public schools to private schools to home-schooling just because you can't really avoid chemicals. I literally looked and felt like I was dying.
>
> High school sucks, I mean most kids don't like high school anyways, but it's even harder when you are known as 'the freak in the corner by the open window with the EpiPen who goes to the hospital a lot.' It was detrimental to my health to even consider going out in public. I would cry in the morning before I had to go to school because it meant that I was going to be in a public place, a public place means lots of people, which means potentially me not coming home. It was that real for me.

Also, on the odd occasion when Tyffanee tried to work in the restaurant, it would usually end up in a trip to the hospital. Inevitably, a customer would come into the restaurant wearing perfume or fragrance and Tyffanee would go into anaphylactic shock, and her throat would swell shut. They almost had an ambulance on standby as she was rushed to emergency so frequently. Tyffanee told me:

> I didn't work very often, and when I did work, it usually resulted in a hospital trip. Customers would come in

WIRED FOR HEALING

*wearing perfumes or cologne or fragrance of any kind. I
didn't really have much of a personal life. I didn't really go
anywhere or do anything. I stayed home most of the time
because it was safe there.*

Her parents took Tyffanee to every doctor that they could
find. They tried an exhaustive list of both allopathic and alternative medical practitioners that could not offer any lasting relief of
her symptoms. This was extremely frustrating and disappointing
for the entire family, but for no one more than Tyffanee:

> *When I went to the specialists, they didn't know what it
> was. They pretty much closed their doors and told me they
> didn't know, so I was on my own. When I went to see the
> allergist, she did a number of different allergy tests, and
> they all came back normal, I guess you could say. She told
> me that this was not an allergy, so she couldn't help me
> either and she didn't know how to treat me.*

Tyffanee was sixteen when she saw a doctor who suggested
that her future was not very promising if her health continued
to decline. She was informed that her lungs were deteriorating
at a rapid rate, but due to her sensitivities, she would not be a
good candidate for a lung transplant. Tyffanee explained:

> *Before, when I had exposure to chemicals, I would go
> into anaphylactic shock. My throat would swell shut, my
> lungs would shut down, I couldn't breathe. I had headaches, I got dizzy, sometimes I'd even get a rash on my
> arms. It was bad. I had to use my EpiPen, go to the hospital, where they'd give me all sorts of steroid injections
> to stabilize my lungs, heart monitors, respirators, oxygen*

masks, antihistamines. My doctors told me that if I lived to see my 30th birthday, it would be a medical miracle. My lungs were rapidly deteriorating, and they even compared giving me a lung transplant to giving an alcoholic a new liver. Because of my chemical sensitivity, my body would just naturally deteriorate any other lungs, so it was like delaying the inevitable. There was no option; there was nothing for me. All I could do was kind of tough it out and make the best of the next 10 years. Telling a sixteen-year-old girl that she has her years numbered is a very harsh thing to hear.

Tyffanee found out about the DNRS through her aunt. She had read an article that I had written for the Kelowna Capital News about my own recovery story from multiple chemical sensitivities and learned that I was now teaching a program to help other people recover. Her aunt told Tyffanee's mom who pleaded with Tyffanee to take the program. But Tyffanee was not so keen on the idea. She was tired of seeking help and didn't want to be disappointed again. She had basically accepted that she was going to die and wanted her mom to come to that acceptance as well. Her mother continued to plead with her, and Tyffanee made a promise to her mother that she would take the program on one condition: when it was over, her Mom would stop pestering her and let her die in peace. In Tyffanee's words:

I didn't want to take the program. I was very skeptical. In fact, when I first heard about it, I laughed and thought, "oh yeah, another con artist trying to get in our pockets." I had already tried everything I could possibly think about doing, and I was so tired of being disappointed that I didn't want to get excited about this working because I didn't want to feel that disappointment again. I thought, if all the doctors that I went to see couldn't figure it out, how can this woman? But she did.

When Tyffanee started the program, she was very fidgety, and I could sense that she really didn't want to be there. I had talked to her on the phone prior to the program to ensure that she was a good candidate; however, by this time I knew that she did not really believe that anyone could help her. I also understood how illness has a way of eating away at hopes and dreams.

But I could see a small flicker of hope returning on the first day of the program. From what I recall, there was a moment of connection when I was telling my own story of what my life was like when I had a limbic system disorder. As I relayed my experience of escalating sensitivities, increased illness, and growing isolation, I could see a light go on for Tyffanee. Perhaps for the very first time, she was actually interacting with someone who had experienced what she was experiencing. Furthermore, I hadn't just *experienced* the illness, I was now recovered. She sat there in a state of disbelief when she heard me describe what she understood as *her* disorder: how it affected her senses, how her body was reacting, and how that influenced her thoughts and feelings. From that point forward, even though she couldn't completely follow along with the neuroscience explanation or fully understand how her brain was not functioning properly, I had her attention. I could sense that she was intrigued but still not completely sold on the idea. However, by the end of the first day, she was feeling more relaxed and was willing to go home and do her homework. When she came in on the second day, we were all in for a bit of a shock.

During the evening of the first day of the program, Tyffanee's sense of smell returned to normal, and she was no longer reacting to fragrances or chemicals! As Tyffanee described it:

Since the first day of the program, I've noticed a lot of changes. Even after the first class, I felt so much better. My sense of smell has changed significantly. I don't smell fragrances as poisons anymore. I smell them for the fragrances that they actually are. I can enjoy the smell. Natural smells, too, I've noticed, flowers even, smell pretty, they don't smell like toxins. And perfumes, as bad as they are, they smell nice now. They smell the way they used to smell. Normal.

Tyffanee cried in joy and disbelief from the beginning of the second day until the last day of the program. She was in absolute shock that her life could turn around so quickly and that now she had the rest of her life to look forward to, without illness. We all cried along with her, for her happiness, for her family and for the new Tyffanee, who could now go out and conquer the world. For Tyffanee it seemed like a miracle. She didn't understand how she changed her condition, she just knew that she did, and she was willing to continue whatever she needed to do to ensure that it would stay that way. On the last day of the program Tyffanee said:

This program changed my life. Now I can go to college, I can go out for dinner, I can go to movie theaters and malls. I can go to parties and to friends' houses. I can be a normal 18-year-old. I feel like I missed so much growing up, being a teenager, but now I feel like I don't have to miss the rest of my life. I can grow into an adult and be normal now. I'm not afraid anymore. I don't have anything to be afraid of. The world is potentially a really cool place, and now I just want to see it all.

During the next six months of her retraining period, Tyffanee did experience a brief episode of returning sensitivities; however, the symptoms were minor in comparison to her reactions before. When this happened, she got scared and thought that maybe her good luck had run out and that perhaps this was just a short-term fix. But with renewed focus on her limbic system rehabilitation practice, the symptoms went away. She is symptom-free to this day and can do anything and go anywhere.

Tyffanee made a comment to me about her recovery process that was quite telling. She noted how we adapt to sickness and also how we adapt to feeling well again:

> At first everything was exciting. I would walk by a body lotion shop, and I was excited because I could smell it, but I wasn't reacting or dying from it. That was great. And then after awhile, I didn't really notice as much. I mean, you don't really know that you just smelled something and didn't react to it. You don't think about it. It just becomes normal. You don't think about the bad things that could have happened that didn't – because they just don't happen. Now I'm just happy in general.

When I asked what advice Tyffanee would give to other people who are still suffering, she said:

> My advice to anybody out there who is struggling is: don't lose hope. Don't give up. Take this program and commit to it. It takes a lot of dedication, but it worked well for me, and it can for you too.

When I asked Tyffanee what advice she would give to people who are already taking the program, she said:

Practise, practise, practise! I practised all day, every day. I practised out loud, in my head, lying down in bed. I practised as much as I could because I figured that if I noticed the slightest change in just one class, then if I practised a lot that, I would be good. I was really committed to the program because I knew that, if I wasn't committed, then it was never going to work. I knew that I had to give it 100% if I was going to make anything of it, if I was going to get any better. And I'm so glad that I did. It's a lot of hard work, but it all boils down to your brain function and changing the way your brain processes things.

When I asked Tyffanee what life is like now she answered:

I don't really think about what it was like to be sick. I forget I was sick sometimes, which is really good – it's amazing actually. And normal is a big change for me. When I was sick, everything revolved around being sick, where I went, who I hung out with, what I did. I virtually didn't go anywhere, or do anything because I was scared. But now I can do everything, and I don't really hesitate anymore. I don't even notice that I ever was sick. It's kind of good to feel normal I guess. The possibilities for my future are endless now. I am definitely going to go to college, but I don't know what I'm going to do with myself yet – everything that I can, I guess.

In the afternoon of the last day of the program, as everyone was sitting politely in their chairs and intently listening to me, Tyffanee was sitting on the floor and using her chair as a table to write on. I thought that she was just taking notes. When the program was over, my associate Candy handed me a letter that was from Tyffanee. Candy told me that Tyffanee didn't want to say goodbye because "good-byes suck and she hates them," but she wanted me to have this letter.

Her letter was neatly folded into squares and sealed with her nametag adorned with lipstick marks where she had kissed it. I didn't open it until later that evening and to this day, I still have her letter in my nightstand beside my bed. Tyffanee wrote:

Dear Annie,

How words escape me when I try and think about how I could ever fully show my gratitude and appreciation for what you have done for me. In the last few days, I want to sing again. Dance again. Live again. And now because of you, I can. You gave me life when I felt like I wanted to die. Showed me light when all I could see is darkness. And most of all, you gave me faith when I thought God had abandoned me. You say you are in the business of witnessing miracles, but Annie, I say from the bottom of my heart, you were my miracle. With everything you've been through, you are still able to help people like myself who need it more than ever. For the first time in my teenage years, I feel alive, and like I want to live. I can feel my dreams and goals flooding back into my reprogrammed brain. I want to go to college, work a normal job, and now more than ever, I want to help people the way you helped me. And with your help, I know I can do it. Thanks for everything you have done, not only for me, and for all of the people you've already helped, but more importantly, thank you for helping the people you will help. I'm sure at some point they will be my friends and family. And you've changed my life, and you will change theirs, too. You are an amazing woman, with the single most amazing heart. I don't need to tell you how lucky you are to have a huge-hearted, loving man beside you while you climb up the ladder of success. On behalf of my friends, my family, I'd like to thank you for giving them "Tyffanee" back. I know that the last five years have given them a hard time, too, but know this: by changing my life, you changed theirs as well. I truly hope there is some way I can help you help others. If ever there is an opportunity for me to do anything to put some faith back in other people's lives, please let me know. From my heart straight to yours. I THANK YOU! You saved a life.

With love,
Tyffanee

Tyffanee did go on to graduate from college. She has a boyfriend, has moved to a new town, and has a new job. We still keep in touch, and twice she has come to our program to speak to the participants. She is very authentic and has a way of genuinely connecting to people from her heart. She has the unique ability to communicate how she is feeling and bravely speaks the words that many are afraid to.

Thank you, Tyffanee, for working so diligently at rewiring your limbic system and for having the courage and wisdom to live your life to the fullest. You have the ability to soften even the hardest of hearts. You make the world a better place, and your story is doing just what you wanted it to do. You are such a huge source of inspiration and hope for many. Thank you for being such a good student and a warrior of the highest degree. The world is truly your oyster!

CHAPTER 13

Stapled to the Couch

Anna had suffered from a number of illnesses related to limbic system imbalance. As the symptoms of depression, anxiety and hypervigilance increased, gradually she changed her life to accommodate her illness. It wasn't a conscious choice, rather, it was based on trying to achieve the best possible quality of life while avoiding the feelings of discomfort or pain. Physically, Anna was suffering from low energy and consistent low-level body pain. She also suffered from a lot of lower back pain and headaches and as a result, she was quite apprehensive about exercising or about other physical activity. She would evaluate situations and make decisions based on terms of energy output costs and potential pain. She also took a fair amount of over-the-counter painkillers.

Anna did not realize that the moderate level of chemical sensitivities that she eventually developed and that the discomfort or pain that she was experiencing were actually symptoms of limbic system dysfunction. Indeed, she didn't know that there was a direct connection between her brain and her state of physical health. As part of her prior diagnosis of depression and anxiety, she understood that she had a chemical brain imbalance. She had been taking antidepressants for eleven years and expected to take them for the rest of her life. She had been to two different psychotherapists for a number of years and as a result, Anna possessed an excellent emotional vocabulary and had a great understanding of her condition and its affect on her. Although therapy was an excellent tool in helping Anna to gain a certain amount of peace of mind and in providing her with coping mechanisms, it did not alleviate the lifelong depression that had become the central theme of her life.

For quite some time Anna experienced anxiety along with depression. Anna is very creative and in her early twenties, she thrived in an atmosphere that allowed her to express that creativity. Although she had lots of friends, and she had lots of fun, she still experienced episodes of anxiety and depression that lasted for a few days and sometimes even for a few weeks.

Part of Anna's 'perfect storm' in developing full-blown limbic system dysfunction happened in the late 1990s when she was working in the film industry. Night shifts and long work hours, combined with the stress and demands of the job proved to be a lethal combination, resulting in exhaustion, migraine headaches, and constant anxiety. This eventually culminated in a 'mini nervous breakdown'. After a long break, and recovering from the film job, Anna started to make a short film of her own. This involved writing the script and writing funding applications. For Anna, the project felt like it had been just a pipedream, until she actually started to make it happen. However, instead of feeling like a dream come true, the project took on the feeling of a *film noir*. Unfortunately, Anna suffered from what felt like a permanent anxiety attack during the whole production.

Anna describes what this experience was like as follows:

For the entire production, I felt frozen like a rabbit caught in the headlights. I eventually completed the film but there was so much unnecessary stress and so little joy in the process. I had thought that creating film and video was my calling in life, but with that project I felt like I had proven myself entirely incapable. It was not long after I shot that film that I started on the antidepressants.

Although I could still function on the medication, I didn't feel good. I felt like I could get myself through another day if I really had to. I was pretty good at hiding it – I don't think people knew how things were for me. I was able to take care of myself, hold down a job, keep my apartment relatively clean – I knew all the signs of depression and made sure they weren't too obvious. I wasn't depressed all the time but regularly enough that it was something I came to plan for.

I got through work and accomplished a number of things but it seemed to take me a lot longer than other people – I had to have recovery time and 'safe' time – which usually consisted of being at home alone for a while, sometimes just for an afternoon, sometimes for a few days at a time. I routinely ignored the phone and isolated myself from people. I had to work up to it to be social.

In 2004, Anna met her partner and for the next few years she was generally okay. There was the new relationship to focus on and that made everything better; in fact, it made Anna want to be better. With a new relationship blossoming, Anna became that much more determined to work out whatever her problems were in therapy. This improved her coping skills, along with her emotional analysis skills. But again, depression was still nagging at her in the background.

After a car accident in 2007, things got a lot worse. Anna goes on to say:

I got more anxious, and eventually I got more sensitive to scents and to sounds. My memory got kind of sketchy. I didn't trust anyone, including myself. After the car accident, I started to have erratic and inappropriate emotional reactions, and my anxiety increased. I started to have episodes of hyper-vigilance where I didn't feel safe, even in my own home.

I was still functional, but I was uncomfortable. I didn't feel like myself. I had a lot of anxiety – not attacks per se, but just general anxiety most of the time. Between my frequent bouts of sadness and feeling unsafe out in the world, I had to really work at getting myself to accomplish things. I had to really push myself to get to work. I had a definite loss of motivation. As things became harder to do – out of fear of anxiety or body pain or whatever, it definitely affected my motivation. The responsibility of work would trigger anxiety so often that, when I did work, I was in a constant state of anxiety. I was chronically underemployed to accommodate my depression and anxiety, and I've consistently hesitated and stopped myself in the face of big projects, potential goals, and achievements. It's like I would get dizzy if I went too far out on a limb. I let that fear hold me back.

It wasn't until Anna was experiencing positive shifts as a result of taking the DNRS program that she realized the symptoms that she was experiencing were rooted in the central nervous system. She describes the physical sensations that she was feeling:

My whole body felt charged – kind of like an adrenalin rush. It wasn't my heart but I felt a physical rush – very uncomfortable – and something I very much associated with anxiety. I realized just recently that I had been having that kind of physical reaction to stress for over 20 years. At times of greater stress, it has provoked, nausea, migraine headaches, chronic neck and shoulder pain, and muscle tightness. After the car accident, I began to have cognitive issues – my memory was affected, and I started to not trust my memory, which made it worse. My quality of life was definitely affected, not so much in terms of where I could go, but rather by my own lack of motivation and the anxiety that was associated with trying to accomplish anything.

With depression, there were times when I was just so sad it felt like I was carrying a weight around. The idea of attempting anything triggered a depressive state that would keep me 'stapled to the couch' – unable to move or motivate myself to do anything. Staying still felt safe, even moving around the house or trying to do housework, I would feel a kind of angst and almost a sense of danger. I was often overwhelmed with sadness. So much so that at times I considered suicide. The idea that my life would be made up of this constant sadness, self-criticism, and fear was too much at times. I never actually got to the planning stages, but it was certainly something I thought about.

In 2009, Anna started to notice that her sense of smell had increased, and she started to dislike a lot of perfumes and laundry detergent scents. By 2011, this had increased and was causing headaches and sometimes inappropriate emotional reactions like confusion, depression, and anxiety. She also started to be mildly sensitive to sound and to startle easily.

By the time Anna stumbled upon the DNRS program in 2012, she was familiar with dealing with depression and anxiety and was pretty much convinced that she would just need to cope with it for the rest of her life.

Anna goes on to say:

I was totally skeptical of the DNRS program. First I was skeptical about it working for depression because that was so different than what the program was normally used for. (How could that possibly work for me?) I understood that my brain chemistry was different than other people's and that I needed the medication that I was on to get through my day-to-day existence. I had already accepted the idea that I had a mental health issue. I expected to be on anti-depressants for the rest of my life and I expected that they would never truly fix the problem.

But when I started to do the DNRS DVD program, I could feel my brain coming up with so many excuses. The kind of reticence I had to making changes was almost palpable and so uncomfortable. I let that stop me sometimes and then of course, that meant that the program wasn't working. Then I kind of fell into a series of self-perpetuating doubts – I totally overanalyzed everything and while practising, I tried to kind of convince myself rationally how the program was going to work – I had done quite a lot of therapy and was very much in the habit of logically working through my emotional issues. So then when the program didn't work as quickly and as brilliantly as it had with all the people in the testimonials and stuff, I blamed the program. It took a long time for me to understand that it isn't about what you know about the program – although that helps you understand why it works – it's the act of doing the practice that makes the changes.

Next Anna describes the first real shift that she noticed that gave her hope that maybe depression didn't have to be a life sentence:

My first big sign of a shift was that I started to trust myself. That was such a huge thing. For so long, I honestly didn't trust myself to do the things I said I would or to do the things I knew were good for me. I remember being so overjoyed when I started to make better decisions for myself – just small things like about my diet or just taking care of myself. Before I would say to myself that I should do whatever – not eat that chocolate, get up from in front of the TV, go for a walk, whatever, and then I would kind of watch myself talk myself out of it. I would often feel sort of detached from myself and watch while I perpetuated the situation with bad food, no exercise, cutting myself off from my friends, and I felt powerless to do anything different. I did that so much that I expected that to happen – more so than making a constructive decision, or taking any kind of step toward self-care.

I knew things were changing when I realized that I was learning to like myself, to care for myself and nurture myself, for my own sake. I knew that was a very big step when I felt like I could trust myself to keep doing that.

Anna goes on to describe what it feels like to be freed from the prison of depression:

I don't feel like depression is my life anymore. I'm not as hesitant or as fearful. If that does come up, I just don't let myself go there – I know that sounds too easy, trust me it wasn't, but as soon as I start to feel any symptoms of that nature, I go practise and it prevents it from happening. The things that scared me before have become practice points to work through with the program.

I feel like the big black holes I used to fall into have

gradually been filled in. I might still trip on the place where the hole was, but it's nowhere near so far to fall, and I get up and keep walking so much faster and easier. We're talking a matter of minutes rather than days. Also those moments happen less and less frequently.

I've also gained a huge appreciation for other people and their issues. Knowing my own baggage gives me a lot more patience and empathy for others with their own stuff, especially around mental health issues. That used to be such a stigmatized word to me, and now I understand it a lot better. I realized that states of being are often temporary and that they fluctuate on a regular basis. I'm not so afraid of that anymore, partly because I just don't get as sad as I used to, but I also know that it isn't a permanent state – I can take myself out of it now. Gradually, I was able to get off the antidepressants, which is totally great. Also I proved to myself that the program worked. Honestly, I wasn't expecting that.

Since doing the program I have started to exercise regularly. There's only been one other time in my life when I've been this consistent with exercise and it feels great. My mood overall has improved a lot. I'm not dragging myself around anymore – I feel good about going out and doing things out in the world, I don't shy away from physical activity or from social events. I have taken on much larger projects in my work that I was too afraid of before. The stress of responsibility at work used to trigger anxiety. My reaction to that kind of responsibility is quite different now – I can calmly go through what needs to be done and then do it. If I do get a bit anxious, I work through it and continue on.

I used to have a real aversion to learning new things. When learning new things in the past, if I didn't pick it up *really quickly and if I wasn't really good at it right away, I would have a stress reaction that would sort of freeze me and stop me from being able to take in any new information. That would turn into anxiety. I could feel the chemical or hormone my body was producing, coursing through my system, and it would take me quite a while to come down off it. Before I identified what was happening, I used to think I had a learning disability or something because I would have such intense reactions and not be able to concentrate or learn.*

I also recognized that I used to skip ahead while reading, a habit that's usually associated with dyslexia. I was so eager to get the information that I wouldn't actually read the whole thing, I'd read the first sentence of a paragraph and then skip a few sentences and then read another and skip a few more, then not know why I didn't understand what I was reading!!

I find I have a much better reaction to new ideas now and a lot more stamina for learning. I don't put as much pressure on myself, and I know to give myself a bit of room to get to know new things. I don't have the same fear or stress reactions. I can concentrate longer, and I have a more level-headed approach to learning.

I've also noticed that I don't have as big a reaction to smells. It didn't ever stop me from going places, but I did have some avoidance coping behaviours happening, like automatically covering my mouth and nose when I walked down the detergent aisle at the super market, or if I encountered someone wearing big perfume or smoking. I don't need to do those anymore. Because of that, I think I go more places more readily. I wasn't aware of consciously stopping myself from going to particular places, but I think that must have affected my choices on some level.

I'm also not so scared in general. I think the hypervigilance made me really cranky in public situations. If I was downtown or in a crowded situation, I would get really negative toward the people around me, and I think that stemmed from a low-grade fear and lacking a feeling of personal safety. I've noticed how much easier it is to be in public and how much more positive my daily interactions are with people.

We already had an amount of environmental concern in our household before scent and chemicals became a health issue, so we still use unscented, non-petroleum, biodegradable laundry detergent, dish soap, shampoo and other personal hygiene products. We use low VOC paint and renovation supplies when necessary, all our cleaners are biodegradable, we use reusable and/or biodegradable bags and food containers, water bottles etc. and we try to cut down the amount of plastic we use in general. I keep my exposures to solvents and other chemicals to a minimum because I know the kind of damage that they can cause, and I certainly don't want to go there again. We off-gassed our new mattress on the porch for two weeks before bringing it into the bedroom. We tend to shop at consignment and second-hand stores a lot – reduce, reuse, recycle. I can't afford it at the moment, but if I could, I would be driving an electric or at least a hybrid car.

Regular chemical or petroleum-based products are permanently damaging to the planet, to all the animals that live on it, including humans, and a lot of the chemicals that we are exposed to on a daily basis can cause brain injury, specifically to the limbic system. Knowing the cause of my illness doesn't mean I'm now invincible – just because I recovered this time doesn't mean I can't get injured again. I do my best to prevent that.

When I asked Anna what she would say to others who are still suffering she replied:

> *Just do it. Don't think about it too hard, just do it. I know that a lot of people have big resistance to doing the program – I know I did. One of the things I've come to realize is that resistance is actually a symptom of the condition. That was really important for me to learn. Once I got hold of that, it helped me to get on with doing the program.*
>
> *There's no difference between the kind of faith a medical doctor expects you to have in their practice of medicine and the kind of faith that you need to have in neuroplasticity for this program to work – because you don't need faith, it's science. It's not a freakin' miracle, it's how the brain works. It's how to work with the brain to recover from these types of illnesses.*
>
> *Imagine the reaction when penicillin was first discovered – I'm sure everyone thought that was magic, but it's not. It was eventually explained, and antibiotics are now used everywhere – in fact, they are now overused (but that's another story). Doing the program takes a little longer than, say, taking a pill everyday, but so far there isn't a pill for limbic system conditions. DNRS is the pill. Do the practice – it'll work. There is no down side.*

CHAPTER 14

Get Your Affairs in Order

Gina could not understand why she was getting so sick — it was all quite mysterious at first. Her symptoms started in 2003 with unexplained headaches that turned into migraines. Despite her best efforts at seeking help, over the next few years her health continued to decline and she developed an expanding list of mysterious sensitivities. She went to see fifty-two doctors including general practitioners, chiropractors, neurologists, and specialists in gastro-intestinal medicine, hormones and thyroid function, who were all unable to determine the cause of her strange illness. Within five years, Gina's symptoms escalated to having seizures and stroke-like symptoms from minute exposures to mould or common chemicals. She became allergic to all but eighteen foods. When she would eat the foods she had become allergic to, it would result in a mysterious paralysis. Although Gina loved her job as a teacher, she eventually had to quit, as she was just too sick to function. Unknowingly, Gina was being exposed to toxic mould in the school where she was teaching.

By October 2007, Gina had become wheelchair-bound. Both Gina and her family thought that she was dying and started to document her health decline in an attempt to convince the school system to remediate the mould problem. She thought that documenting her suffering might prevent someone else from the same ill fate. Her condition had worsened to the point that small concentrations of mould in any environment caused seizures or loss of motor skills that would result in paralysis that would last up to two days.

One day, after having a prolonged seizure that was triggered by a well-known glass cleaner, the doctors at the hospital told her husband to "get her affairs in order." They did not have any answers and feared the worst. Although Gina did not pass away, her health continued to deteriorate and the sensitivities and debilitating reactions that resulted from any exposure to mould happened more frequently. She was advised to start wearing a respirator at that point. With the respirator, Gina was able to circumvent the symptoms triggered by mould, however her sensitivities had also increased to other stimuli and she was violently reacting to perfume, cologne, chlorine, and the blue cleaner used in restaurants. Although the respirator seemed to help protect her from mould exposures, it did not circumvent the day-to-day exposures that were now commonplace. Within minutes of any chemical exposure, Gina would crumble to the ground like a rag doll, totally helpless to stop the impending seizure or paralysis. This cycle repeated itself hundreds of times over the period of illness.

Gina was finally diagnosed with toxic encephalopathy that was caused from the toxic mould exposure by doctor #53. Along with the myriad of severe sensitivities she was experiencing, she was also suffering from worsening cognitive decline. Gina could not comprehend simple math. Not unlike stroke patients, she also could not process simple words, her memory was severely affected, she had poor balance and she could not comprehend time or location. For example, she could see the President's face, but she could not remember his name. She knew what day it was, but she did not know whether it was a.m. or p.m. She was unable to remember the current month or year.

With the help of doctor #53, Gina detoxified the mould. This helped restore her cognitive function to a degree, but she was still very sick. She thought that if she removed the mould, that her body would take care of everything else. Yet, seventy-five different types of therapies later, she was still reacting to minute amounts of mould and chemicals.

Gina ordered the Dynamic Neural Retraining System™ DVD program in October of 2011. Within three weeks of starting the program, her sense of smell started to normalize and for the first time in years, she was able to go to a restaurant with her friends — without a respirator. Within one month, symptoms of chronic pain that she thought were unrelated to limbic system impairment also started to disappear. Her energy levels were increasing and she was experiencing better sleep.

Gina understood that she had experienced an acquired toxic brain injury, and that this injury needed to be addressed in a very specific way. She realized that during trauma, her brain had rewired itself in an attempt to protect her from future harm and as a result, her life was being controlled by a maladapted limbic system. Gina referenced her limbic system impairment as 'the beast'. Through the program, she learned how to remap this rogue system that enabled her brain and body to shift out of a state of survival and into a state of growth and repair.

Gina was amazed at the improvements that she was making. For the first time in years, she was able to celebrate Mother's Day with her daughters in public. She attended her daughter's graduation ceremony. She was able to travel long distances and assist her sister in caring for her elderly mother when her mother was unexpectedly admitted to hospital — all huge and unexpected accomplishments for Gina.

After one year, Gina had posted to the DNRS online community forum to report her status.

Gina says:

I am going to pursue part time employment because I choose to. My energy has increased significantly. In addition, I am contemplating taking classes to become an herbalist or clinical nutritionist. It is grand to have options!

It has been said that knowledge is power. I submit to you that knowledge is power when it is acted upon. If you are wondering whether the DNRS Program will work for you, consider your options. If you're like most of us, you have exhausted all of them and are back to square one or worse.

Annie, thank you for embracing your healing journey and in so doing helping others, who like yourself were suffering from very misunderstood illnesses. You helped me (re)train the beast, regain my health, and reclaim my life. I thank you and will forever be grateful.

CHAPTER 15

Alone in the Dark

Linda is from a small town in Alberta, Canada. She is a quiet, humble, and soft-spoken woman with a heart of gold. She is not a woman of many words (much like my own mother) and is not prone to showing a great deal of emotion. She also does not talk about her past very much, and for good reason.

Linda was really unsure if her story would help anyone, as she doesn't consider herself a very special person. Linda does not give herself credit for being brave and strong and for having a sense of faith that is undeniably stronger than most.

Linda has endured more pain and suffering in her life than any human being should ever have to endure. She is brave and courageous beyond measure and has graciously never identified herself with her past or illness. Even in the face of indescribable pain and suffering, she never thought about giving up. She merely accepted that this was the life that she had been given, and she continued to place her faith in God.

Linda knows the path of loneliness and suffering and of the isolation that goes hand in hand with severe environmental illness, and her wish is that her recovery can give someone else hope. I'm certain that her story will not only give you hope, but will also inspire you and will demonstrate Linda's personal strength along with her unshakeable faith.

Linda was sixty years old when she attended the Dynamic Neural Retraining System™ program and had been suffering from severe chemical sensitivities, electric hypersensitivity syndrome, and metal sensitivities since 1980. She took the program in 2011, and for those of you who are doing the math, that means that she had been suffering for 31 years.

In the beginning, Linda developed sensitivities to chemicals. At first, she was only sensitive to chemicals found in cleaning products, paint, wood stains, perfumes, and laundry products. She would start to cough and have a hard time breathing, and her eyes would water.

Linda had suffered a toxic trauma from the chemicals involved in building and remodeling homes. Although Linda's husband was a full time police officer, on the side he and Linda would build homes from scratch, and/or fix them up, and sell them. They had built or renovated and sold eight or nine houses when Linda started to exhibit symptoms of chemical sensitivities. Eventually Linda's sensitivities increased, and her symptoms worsened with time. She noticed at one point that her hair dye was causing the same reactions, so she stopped dying her hair. Her sense of smell heightened, and she could smell the toxic smell of chemicals in any product and also taste them. It felt like she was being poisoned.

Linda's chemical sensitivities progressed from a minor cough to symptoms that affected her entire body. Little did Linda know, this was just the beginning of a thirty-one year nightmare.

Of course, when Linda started to exhibit symptoms of chemical sensitivities, she went to her family doctor, whose only advice was to avoid whatever was making her sick. Linda tried desperately to avoid chemicals; however, this was next to impossible.

True to a toxic trauma that causes limbic system dysfunction, Linda's sensitivities began to spread. Linda also became sensitive to metal. Contact with anything made of metal would cause an array of debilitating symptoms. She could even taste it when she was exposed to metal. Again, in an attempt to avoid what was making her sick, she could no longer eat with metal utensils, cook with metal pots or pans, wear jewelry, or be around anything that contained metal. To avoid metal, Linda would use plastic utensils or CorningWare for cooking. Her husband actually built her a pair of wooden eye glasses as she could no longer wear glasses that had metal frames or contained any metal at all. She also could not sit on a regular chair, as it contained metal springs. She could no longer sleep on her bed because of the metal in the mattress, so she slept on the floor.

After Linda developed metal sensitivities in 1996, she travelled all the way from Alberta to Dallas, Texas to see an environmental doctor and was hopeful that this costly venture would help her. Even the doctors there were perplexed by her symptoms and sensitivity to metals. They did a battery of tests when Linda arrived – one of which was to measure heavy metals. Although this test came back a little higher than normal, they didn't see any reason to do chelation treatments at that time. According to Linda, her treatment at the clinic consisted of intravenous vitamin therapy, allergy shots, exercise, sauna, and a recommendation to avoid the things that caused her symptoms. So Linda returned home and continued to sleep on the floor. Her symptoms continued to get worse and to spread to other stimuli.

In 1998, Linda's 20-year-old daughter Shannon, who had Down syndrome, was diagnosed with leukemia. In 2000, at the young age of 22, sadly Shannon passed away. Linda told me that when Shannon was dying that she told her Mom, "Don't worry about me. I'll be perfectly fine. I'm going to heaven, so, don't worry about me." Shannon was wise beyond her years and always had a sense of purity and innocence about her. Linda goes on to explain, "Having Down syndrome came with a simplicity of love, and Shannon accepted people for who they were – it was quite beautiful really." Understandably, Linda and John, her husband of 30 years, were devastated by the loss of their daughter.

They moved on with life in the best way that they could. They were still under an incredible amount of stress with Linda's declining health. Linda and her husband had very strong faith and adapted to Linda's sensitivities and coping mechanisms. They had come to a place of acceptance of Linda's illness and believed they had done all they could in terms of treatment options.

In a very sad twist of fate, Linda's husband John became suddenly ill in 2003 and was diagnosed with stomach cancer. He passed away six weeks later – he was only 55. During this time Linda found comfort in her faith and her church.

One day after her husband's death, Linda was in the church where they happen to be doing renovations that involved a lot of metal scaffolding. She was in the church for an extended period of time during which she was exposed to a lot of metal. Later that day, she started to get chills and started shaking. She basically spent the next three days curled up in a ball, in severe pain with a burning feeling from head to toe. From that point onward, her sensitivities to metal became extreme and Linda also developed sensitivities to electromagnetic fields (EMFs), like wireless networks or electricity of any kind.

When exposed to the electromagnetic fields that are common in appliances or wireless technology, Linda would experience excruciating pain and other unexplainable symptoms. When she was exposed, she would also suffer from debilitating exhaustion. She was also experiencing a lot of abdominal bloating and "acid reflux burning sensation" in her stomach.

At one point, Linda went to see a naturopath who said that she had extensive food sensitivities and put her on a very restricted diet. However, that didn't help with Linda's symptoms. She also noticed that her heart was beating irregularly – sometimes it would seem to skip a beat. She did see a heart specialist at one time, but the test results were inconclusive.

Linda describes the symptoms in her central nervous system with exposure to electromagnetic fields or metal this way:

> At first, I would get really cold and get the chills and get shaky, and I could taste metal in my mouth. When it progressed, when I was exposed to EMFs, I would get burning throughout my whole body and my nervous system. My skin and every nerve in my body would feel like I was walking on coals. I would get numbness and tingling and burning that affected my entire body. It would just hurt and tingle in pain, almost like a severe sunburn. I also experienced a lot of brain fog and memory problems. You know, trying to think about words because you knew what the word was and you couldn't come up with it.

Linda goes on to describe the sensations of fullness in her head:

> There would be times you'd almost feel like there was pressure. You had pressure coming from within your brain. It just felt like your brain hurt. It just felt like you had an egg-beater going on in your head, which is kind of a whirling, it's a really hard thing to explain, but that's the only way I could explain it. You could always hear it, and it was a horrible feeling. I mean, I know it sounds kind of weird, but that's the only way I can kind of explain it. It just felt like the pressure was coming not from the outside but from the inside.

Linda had also noted that if she was around chemicals that she had a heightened sense of smell and taste. For example, if she was exposed to perfumes or paint, she could taste them.

Here Linda describes what it was like when the illness was at its worst:

> I basically lived with my electricity shut off. I'd have 1 light on in my family room so everything else would be dark, and I'd have to cook without metal utensils or pots. It got to the point where I couldn't go out anywhere because everywhere you went there was the EMF problem, so my remaining daughter would have to get my groceries and do my shopping. Also, because of the metal sensitivities, the furnace ducts would bother me. I couldn't sit over them, or my bed couldn't be over them. I ended up sleeping on the floor in my bathroom. That's the safest place I found.

Linda's life became very restricted and isolated as a result, and eventually she lost most of her friends. As her sensitivities escalated, Linda found it more and more difficult to have anyone in her home. She describes it like this:

> If people came to visit me, they could not bring their cell phones with them or have chemicals of any kind on them, like their laundry detergent or personal hygiene products. So it got to the point where it was becoming too hard to be a friend because I couldn't go anywhere or do anything. And so I was dropped by a lot of my friends. On the odd occasion, if someone did come to visit, and I let them in the house with chemicals or metal on them, I would be sick for a minimum of three days afterwards. I would get a lot of

nerve pain and get the chills inside where no matter what I did – I just couldn't get warm. I was cold all the time. Along with the 'egg-beater head' feeling, I just basically felt really unwell. There was one couple that did come to visit me and were very great in accommodating my special needs. They would sit in the dark with me if needed. They would mow my lawn for me because they knew that I couldn't do it myself. But most people just dropped off.

Linda was also limited in terms of using a telephone. Cell phones were definitely out of the question. Cordless phones were also not an option. Even using a regular corded phone caused reactions. Occasionally Linda would talk on a speakerphone, but even that caused symptoms.

Linda had to severely alter the way that she lived, even inside her home. She tried to make her house as safe as possible. She basically shut off all the circuit breakers so that there was no electricity. She could not sit on any furniture that contained metal or that had metal springs or metal legs. The only piece of furniture that she had that did not create symptoms was a wooden chair that she placed in a specific spot in her kitchen.

Linda was so severely affected by electromagnetic fields and all electronics that she could not watch TV or listen the radio or CDs. If she tried, it would result in debilitating pain. During the evenings, Linda sat alone in her house, in the dark, in a wooden chair in her kitchen, in silence. She could not even have a burning candle as the smell of natural candles was making her sick.

When I asked Linda what got her through this dark time of her life, she said it was her faith in God. She never thought of killing herself although the idea of simply disappearing or crawling into a safe corner somewhere had appeal. But there was no safe place for her. Linda describes this time in her life:

In order to try to avoid all the triggers in my life, I had to isolate myself from everyone and everything. I basically just stayed in my own home. I couldn't go anywhere, couldn't go shopping, and couldn't go get groceries, go to the bank, or do anything. I just lived in my house. I had to have most of the power shut off. So it was quite dark, I had no TV. No radios. I seldom talked on the phone – and if I did it was for a short time on a speakerphone. And basically, when it was wintertime, I sat in the dark. I couldn't use candles. So it was basically sitting in the dark and doing nothing. And that's how I had to live my life.

Leaving the house at all required a lot of planning in advance and involved trying to avoid all of the potential triggers, which were endless. Walking or driving anywhere required knowledge about where the power lines were or the cell phone towers in order to avoid them. Even when she went to her doctor's office, he would have to get a wooden chair for Linda and meet her in a room in the back of the clinic that had tiled flooring as Linda was reacting to the finish on the hardwood floors.

In the summer when the weather was good enough to leave the house, Linda would go for a walk, but had to be very careful with where she walked. For example, she couldn't walk on a pathway beside a metal fence, as that would cause symptoms. She couldn't be around any power lines or cell phone towers. She had found one small section of a path that worked for her. Occasionally, a friend would join her and they would walk back and forth on just that section of the path.

Then she discovered DNRS:

I took the program in March of 2011. I found out about the program from a friend of mine who had the same challenges as I had with EMF and chemicals, and she used to live in the area that I live in and moved to the coast because she wanted to be in a safe environment. And she found out from a friend of hers, who knew Annie when Annie was sick and was challenged in her life. And then she found out that Annie was better and that she had created this program for people to recover like she did. So my friend, Karen, went to the program and she, amazingly, got so much better after the program that I thought "yes, this is something that will work for me, and I'm going to do it." So that's what I did.

Even attending the program was a huge challenge for me. Friends of mine, the same ones that came to sit with me in the dark, drove me there, and we had to go on a ferry and had to try to find some accommodations that would be safe for me. So I'd rented a house on the ocean and that way I could control my environment better. So that's what we did.

We drove in the one day. We got up, and we left here at 4 a.m. and drove the whole way because I couldn't stop at a hotel or anything, so we had gone the whole way and had to take the ferry, whatever. Had to plan all that out and get there all in one day. The house actually did work fine because the lady that owned it was chemically sensitive so that part was good, and they had wireless there so we just unplugged it, and basically, it was good. I had a wooden portable bed, and I brought it along so I could sleep on that, so it all worked out.

I didn't notice any big shifts during the program, like some others do. The recovery period for me was a little longer than most people. It took me about ten months before

I really had a big shift. After completing the course, I did have small changes, and it was slow, but it was still steady. But I had my big shift in about ten months time after I had taken the course. But I continued to practise everyday. I practised an hour in the morning and a half hour in the evening before I went to bed. I also practised any time that I was feeling challenged, which was a lot. And I was determined that the program would work, and I knew it would work because it had already worked for my friend Karen. And I just continued. I think it's important that people do that – not to give up and to keep on going and know that the program works. I remember the time when Candy had said, "if you keep on practising, your brain has no choice but to rewire, so I thought, "yes, I'm just going to continue on, and it happened. And it's good – you have to do the practice.

Linda goes on to talk about her big 'aha!' moment during her recovery:

A big turning point for me was when my brother-in-law passed away. I really wanted to go, and I wanted to be there for my sister. So I drove there, and I was sitting outside the church, and I was thinking to myself, "I can't go in there. I don't think I can go in there. I don't think I can do this. There are too many cell phones, and then there's the big sound system." And I thought, "well, Linda, that's silly. You can go in. It's the fear that's holding you back." And I realized that on the drive there, I had been trying to convince myself that I wasn't ready for that yet. That it was too big of a challenge for me. Then it suddenly dawned on me, "it's the fear! It's the fear that's stopping me!" So,

I just said, "that's silly," and I walked into the church, and I was fine. Then the next morning, I had to do one of the readings at the front, with a microphone, and I was fine. I didn't have any symptoms.

I basically realized that my life has changed because now I could just go anywhere I wanted, and basically after that, it just got better and better and better. And you know, I still do think, years later, that things still continue to get better. Even though I was still having some symptoms, they weren't as large as what I was having before. They were considerably less. And I didn't have that fear. It was fear that was keeping me from accepting the positive changes that I was already making.

I asked Linda to elaborate on how she could rationalize still having symptoms with her recovery process. She said that instead of going to fear, she would use any exposure as an opportunity to rewire her brain. This is how Linda describes it:

Well, because the symptoms were less than what I was getting before, I just knew that every time I exposed myself, I realized, "I'm just re-wiring my brain every time I come in contact with something," and then it just kind of melts away. And then every time I went out somewhere, it got less and less and less, and pretty soon I didn't even notice. I'd drive somewhere, and there was a telephone tower, well, I'd even forgotten it was there. Then I'd think, "well, I'm just normal now."

I attended the program, and it was amazing. It changed my life completely. And being with other people in the group was really helpful and supportive and I think that the facilitators were so helpful with answering questions and just knowing that they, too, had been sick and gotten better was a really big part of how successful the program is.

Before attending the DNRS program, I went to a naturopath, and I saw two environmental health doctors. I went all the way to Dallas to the environmental health clinic. And still I was sick. I continued to get sicker actually. I ended up going to a naturopath and, of course, they did testing and gave some kind of drops that they said might help. I can't recall the name of them, but it didn't help. And then I had gone to see another environmental health doctor, and he has this program, and he does a bunch of blood work, urinalysis, and it's all sent away down to the States. At that time, it cost $5,000 just for that. And the tests came back that I had high heavy metals and different things like that. But the environmental doctor could not explain the symptoms because he had seen others with levels of heavy metals that were way higher than me that didn't have as many or as severe symptoms as me. I did do chelation treatments for heavy metals, but that didn't work either. Their only advice beyond all of the treatments that they were recommending was avoidance.

Some of the things I can do now that I wasn't able to do in the past are pretty much everything. I can do anything! Things like mowing my grass. I could never in a million years before, mow my grass. Number one, the smell of the grass and the gas, but also the mower contained something metal that I had to be pushing around which I couldn't do before. And so I'm quite joyful to be able to go out and cut my grass. I can go out for dinner. I can fly on an airplane. I can go to an airport. I can go to church. I can go out for dinner with my friends. I can have people in. They can have their cell phones. I can sit on anything. I can use an iPAD. I can listen to music or watch TV. I can watch a movie or do whatever. I can go out with my family, my grandchildren, and you know, watch a movie with them.

It just feels... it's amazing. It really is. Because when you're taken away from them and can't do anything with your family, it really hurts. My grandchildren used to say things like, "oh well, you know, Gram can't go there, Gram can't do this" or "she can't do that" and now I can! I just feel so much more part of their lives it's wonderful!!

The first time I went out with them, they took me out for lunch at the Cheesecake Café, and they said, "Well Gram, we can't believe we're actually sitting in a restaurant! You're here, you can do this!" You know, and I'm using metal utensils, and every time that I accomplished something, they would join in on the celebration really. So it didn't just affect my life, it affected my family and friends, too.

The first time I got on an airplane, I was very excited, and also a bit nervous. A bit apprehensive, I guess, because that was a huge challenge. But yeah, I just focused on my iPad, and it was totally fine. I just felt so much joy that... it was wonderful. I don't know, I can't explain it. It's beyond words in many ways.

I actually got a laptop, which is kind of cool. I can Skype – I'm on Facebook. I can use a cellphone. I can drive anywhere I want to drive no matter if there are power lines or cell towers. I can vacuum. I can cut my own grass – which is amazing for me because I couldn't do that before. I can go to a restaurant. I can go to someone's house. I can go into anybody's vehicle. I can use utensils that are made from metal, and I can cook in metal. I can use anything I want to use, which is wonderful! And my life is just amazing now *because there are no restrictions. It's wonderful! Basically, I can go anywhere I want to go and do anything I want to do.*

In terms of electromagnetic radiation, I do respect the research that has been done in this area, and I accept that it can be unhealthy. I still would not live in a wireless situation maybe 24/7 because that's something that I choose to do. But if I'm going out, and there's WIFI around, I think it's perfectly fine, too. It's out there. I think if we use it in moderation then it's perfectly fine.

I asked Linda what she would say to others who are still suffering?

It's really hard to put into words what the program has done for me. It just changes your life in such an amazing way, and knowing that all your hard work of getting to that point is worth it because life is worth it.

I would say that there is hope and to take the program because you cannot believe how much it actually changes your life. I mean, people I know are skeptical because they've tried so many different things, but this is something totally different, and it's the only way to recover. That no matter what they have to do, to go and take the course somewhere because you just have to totally believe and trust and try something totally different because they won't have to suffer anymore. They can go on and lead a normal life.

If you are sick right now, I encourage you to take the program because it will change your life completely. You will get better. It is an amazing program and please – have the courage to do it and no matter what your time limit is in recovery, it will work. Just be patient and keep on practising. You won't get any better if you don't practise consistently. And that's essential. It totally is. And change will happen. It may not be in three days or three months or whatever, but I think if you stick to it, it'll work, it'll happen.

I know how it feels to be so desperate and not know how you're going to manage the next day – to be so lonely because you can't be around people. There is hope, there really truly is. The program works. So I encourage you to do it.

In the fall of 2013, Linda went to Disneyland with her grand-children. From living in the dark to hanging out with Mickey Mouse! Gram can truly do anything!

CHAPTER 16

From Healthy to Disabled in One Year

This chapter is written directly by a participant who wrote about the progression of her illness and subsequent recovery. Thank you, Linda, for your wisdom and for documenting your recovery.

LINDA W. – 2011/2012

"Never take good health for granted!" This has been my mantra for most of my adult life.

Could a woman be active, energetic, and healthy one year, and then almost bed-ridden with debilitating medical problems the next? I would not have thought so, being blessed with good health most of my life, running my own small business, living with my husband and two poodles in our lovely log home, taking five- to fifteen-mile hikes in the Maryland mountains, entertaining friends, and traveling whenever and wherever I wished. But suddenly, everything changed.

Through a combination of factors, including stress, I developed multiple chemical sensitivities (MCS), electromagnetic field sensitivity (EMFS), and chronic fatigue syndrome (CFS), beginning in the spring of 2009 and reaching my physical and emotional bottom by the summer of 2010. By July of that year,

I was barely able to function although I forced myself to get up in the morning, dress, walk my poodles, and more or less keep going until early afternoon when I would go back to bed for the rest of the day.

To summarize, under life's stresses and my reaction to them, my autoimmune system broke down. Then the amygdala, the gland that responds to stress and danger, went into over-drive, secreting excess adrenalin and reacting to everything as a threat of equal magnitude. This resulted in multiple hypersensitivities and a multitude of symptoms. I became uncharacteristically fearful and anxious; the adrenal gland sensing my fear, re-doubled its efforts to warn me of danger (Fight! Flight!) – a vicious cycle had begun. For some sufferers, these issues come from exposure to a virus, an overload of toxins, or other environmental factors, or from psychological causes. There is debate in medical scientific communities about the origins, causes, and dynamics of such profound events, but agreement among those who experience them is that they are life-changing and challenging in the extreme.

I first became reactive to certain plastics, specifically those used to manufacture water bottles, and to all products made from recycled water bottles (Polar Fleece, some commercial packaging, some vehicle interiors, selected medical devices, plastic grocery bags, etc.). This plastic is polyethylene terephthalate; the terephthalate, which is used to make plastics flexible, is a known toxin. I developed hives, rashes, bruises, and almost unbearable itching. Cold showers and anti-itch creams and lotions helped only a little. Ultimately, I was placed on two antihistamines, twice a day, which brought some relief.

This situation remained just manageable until the winter of 2010 when we were buried under 70 inches of blowing, drifting snow on our mountain. I was in an enclosed space with plastics and electronics almost 24/7, and the sensitivities bloomed. By spring, I was sick; by summer, I was desperate.

I was reacting to electromagnetic fields, which include cell phones, WiFi, cordless phones, computers, handheld devices, lights (most especially florescent lights) and light sockets, TV, DVD players, telephones and jacks, microwave ovens, microwave and cell phone towers, overhead power lines, and ambient electromagnetic fields in the atmosphere around me. The symptoms included a crushing headache, terrific pressure on my chest, blurred vision, and a generalized feeling of illness, coupled with fear and anxiety, as the adrenalin coursed through my body.

During this time, I developed every symptom associated with CFS. These include depression, erratic blood sugar, inability to focus, short-term memory loss, insomnia, inability to taste accurately, weight loss, muscle pain throughout my body, and an extreme, unceasing fatigue.

My internist, an allergist, and a specialist at Johns Hopkins Hospital were baffled and unable to help me. I had tests I had never heard of and tried medications that often made me feel worse.

I believe in the power of prayer. All through this ordeal, friends and friends of friends prayed; my own prayers usually consisted of "Help." I didn't ask "Why?" I believe that some things are given to us to pass on our experience, knowledge, and hope to others. The priority was how to stop the deadly progression before it caused neurological damage. I battled self-pity, refusing to assume the role of a Poor Me victim, I discarded toxins, pulled plugs from the walls... anything to keep things from getting worse.

It is known that 80% of the spouses of people with these sensitivities leave! My husband stood by me, suffering agonies of concern and fear for my health and my sanity – and for my survival. He was uncomplaining about this retro-lifestyle of primitive lighting and limited communication. Together, we rediscovered books. Friends called, wrote, and visited briefly, dispensing hugs and supporting me with their love. My website clients stayed with me, patiently waiting as I worked on their sites for only one hour in the morning – my absolute limit on a computer, and only on a laptop.

At the low point in this progression, July 2010, we had hard-wired phones: my daughter and her partner came from the UK and, being an innovative and resourceful women, rewired the phone lines to the outside of the house, bypassing all the jacks. Our electrician spent many hours in our home, helping me to identify all the breakers, turning off many and re-wiring others to relieve my discomfort while maintaining some semblance of normalcy in our lives. We had only essential electricity. I slept in a 'clean' space, totally devoid of all electricity within the room or nearby. We became connoisseurs of unscented candles and little book-lights, which, when snapped to the front of our belts, made us look like fireflies in reverse moving through our darkened house at night or on cloudy days. We bought a tiny AM/FM battery-powered radio to keep in touch with the outside world. If the speaker was facing away from me, I could tolerate this radio for a limited period of time. I could talk on the phone for about ten minutes, after which I would begin to lose my voice and remaining strength. I tried a speakerphone, but that caused pain. At my request, our local power company sent technicians to check the breaker box and to scan the underground cables for any leaks or breakage; all was in order, eliminating possible issues in that area. They also reassured me that I could safely walk over the buried lines in our yard; the lines were buried very deeply and did not cause me pain or danger. I could, however, feel the emissions from a close neighbor's powerful satellite TV.

My Hyundai SUV was completely lined with recycled plastics and strong electronics, so we purchased a much less toxic Honda CR-V so that I could once again be driven to the grocery store, where my husband did most of the shopping and checked out, while I fled the chemicals and electricity in the building to wait outside. Even in this improved vehicle, I rode wrapped like a mummy in scarves and shawls to protect me from toxicity that I could feel burning my skin. I spent a few hours each day in a tiny cabin I had purchased years ago and placed in the meadow behind our house. Only now did the true purpose of this seemingly frivolous whim become clear: It was now my sanctuary, completely clear of all my 'enemies.' I lay in a lounger since I could not sit up for more than a few minutes. I had many blankets, pillows, and books for comfort and company. Then I received a call from Carol.

Carol is a woman of enormous courage, with a dramatic personal history of MCS and with a mission: she seeks out and offers to help those of us who suffer similar afflictions. Carol gave me a key suggestion: "You might try getting rid of all the chemicals in your house…" – so simple, so obvious (although not to me), and ultimately, so effective. My husband and I filled trash bags with cleaning products, laundry and dishwashing liquids, waxes, etc., etc. – it is amazing how many chemicals abide in a house, creating a toxic stew even for those without obvious sensitivities. For me, they were deadly. Within a day, I began to feel less uncomfortable, to breath more easily, to feel less oppressive fatigue. I replaced the essentials with white vinegar and water sprays and with Seventh Generation products, a very low-toxicity line of dish, laundry, and cleaning items. A friend without sensitivities visited and said, without prompting, "It feels better in here – have you changed something?" I had been given another clue to the mystery of my healing.

After trying other neuroplasticity-based programs, I had reached a plateau in my healing process. I then investigated a program for brain retraining called the Dynamic Neural Retraining System (www.dnrsystem.com) that was mentioned in an inspiring article in the New York Times one Sunday. This program was designed and implemented by a woman named Annie Hopper who had been afflicted by several of these hypersensitivities. She was a trained therapist and, therefore, was able to determine that her hypersensitivities were brain-related and to devise a method of addressing the entire limbic system of the brain to alter and normalize its responses to perceived stimuli. At this very moment in time, when I was searching for further help, Annie Hopper released a set of DVDs, incorporating sessions from a three-day seminar that she offers in various cities in the US and Canada. As I was still unable to travel, I ordered the DVDs and began to work this program.

To summarize briefly, Annie Hopper's approach to hypersensitivities of the sorts that I have experienced is to consider the entire limbic system of the brain – the amygdala, the hypothalamus, and the hippocampus – and to activate areas in the frontal lobe. Her program requires daily exercise and practice every day for six months. The DVDs illustrate the reasoning behind this intense, repetitive practice, which is based on solid scientific facts and constantly evolving knowledge, and they show the seminar in progress as well as inspiring testimonials on the final day from the participants. She suggests several books that are relevant to this brain work, one of which, *The Brain That Changes Itself* by Dr. Norman Doidge, is reason enough to offer hope to anyone with any brain-related issues. I plan to read others on her list as well.

One of the great positives to the Dynamic Neural Retraining System is the availability of assistance and support online and by phone. Annie Hopper and her assistants have set up an online 'community' where registered members are encouraged to post their progress toward healing from their many hypersensitivities and to ask for help regarding points about which they are uncertain. The supportive and positive atmosphere on that forum is invaluable, especially to someone who cannot attend live seminars. I have benefited immensely in the two weeks that I have been working with this system.

One of the many short-term goals of the program is to expand one's capabilities in the presence of 'triggers' that have, in the past, resulted in massive overreactions in the limbic system. In my two weeks work, I have activated two additional breakers in the house and have ridden in a vehicle that is the twin of the one that I was obliged to sell due to my intolerable reactions to it, with virtually no reaction.

The program is based on the premise that six months of dedicated and diligent work with the exercises and gradual, intelligent expansion of one's life-boundaries will be the key to complete healing. I am absolutely willing to invest as much time as necessary to achieve this prize. My journey continues!

PROGRESS! – MARCH 2012

I have been working with the Dynamic Neural Retraining System™ program for just over three months. In that short time, I have begun to see exciting progress. One of the keys to this, in my belief, is Annie Hopper's gentle but firm insistence on expanding one's 'comfort zone' by gradually increasing exposures and decreasing avoidance behaviours, using the program in a mindful and intelligent way. The other major factor in my progress has been the forums on the DNRS web site which are overflowing with accounts from people working the program in all sorts of situations which would have challenged them intolerably in the past and which they are now coming through victoriously.

I have committed to six months of daily practice as well as to applying the program in every situation that causes significant symptoms, day to day. We now have most of the normal electricity on full time in the house with no effect on my body. I am able to tolerate some chemicals, too, although I tend to steer clear of intense smells and notably toxic things, which seems more like common sense than avoidance to me!

My most dramatic victory to date was spending time in an airport waiting for friends to arrive. I have always loved the bustle and kinetic energy of airports but was unable to tolerate the powerful electricity and many chemicals there for years now. In January, I was able to wait comfortably, working the program in my mind when I felt a reaction begin; the reactions faded away. I was filled with gratitude and joy!

I was able to achieve my primary short-term goal: I watched the Westminster Kennel Club dog show on satellite TV – and saw my daughter, with her camera, working the ringside! Next goal, a train trip, sometime in the not-too-far distant future – and of course, the remaining breakers in our house!

Most days are not dramatic, most changes are subtle, but they add up to the picture of a woman returning to 'normal,' rejoining life. I continue to use Annie's method, with steady, gratifying, and life-giving results. I owe my life to these wise and innovative people who are forging new trails through the dark maze of pain, fear, and confusion that is life with extreme sensitivities.

Hope is a precious gift; thank you Annie, for the gift of hope! Onward!

This is my six-month anniversary! I committed to the DRNS program for six months, and I have achieved that goal with astonishing results, some of which I planned and some of which came as surprises.

I had begun to experience significant improvement in my reactions to chemicals and electromagnetic fields and stress by the middle of March, my three-month point (see above). During the three months since my mid-point update, I had continued to work on expanding my tolerance, turning on more breakers in the house, shopping in more stores, having company for lunch – 'normal' life pleasures. I had, as my next goal, a trip somewhere. "Be careful what you ask for!"

Unexpectedly, in March, my husband became an urgent candidate for heart valve replacement surgery. There was no question that we would agree to this, as we have a fine cardiologist, and we had known that this procedure would be needed some day... the sudden urgency was the surprise. We began the complex series of steps required to prepare for his surgery at Johns Hopkins Hospital in Baltimore. On March 22nd, our 32nd anniversary, we spent the day at the hospital while Tom ran the gauntlet of pre-op tests. We spent the night in a very comfortable all-suites hotel a few blocks from the hospital. At 5:30 the next morning, the hotel shuttle delivered us to the door of Johns Hopkins again, and Tom was prepped and taken into surgery. His son and I waited together, and six hours later we were allowed to see Tom in the cardiac ICU. Thus began a two-week adventure, as Tom progressed through various nursing units and stages toward discharge, which came on Easter Sunday when I carefully drove him home.

As I reread that paragraph, I am forcefully struck by the simplicity of my words: "spent the night in a hotel," "waited in the hospital," "two weeks later." But these are profound statements. To those who have not experienced MCS, EHS, or CFS, staying in a hotel for multiple nights, spending days in a huge hospital as a loved one recovers, and driving distances are 'What you do.' To me, unable only a few short months before to tolerate even a fraction of the toxins and powerful assaults found in either of those places, and the attendant stress, and to manage the two-hour drive each way on days when I did not stay at the hotel, would have been, without question, impossible.

Before we went to Hopkins, I doubled down on my brain work, focusing on what I knew would be challenging circumstances. Then, on March 22nd, I threw myself on God's mercy, put my trust in DNRS and went for it!

I experienced a miracle! During the entire time in Baltimore and 'commuting' from home, I experienced only very slight twinges of itching and what I believe was probably normal fatigue for anyone in this situation. I was able to sleep well, eat heartily, and support Tom and concerned friends who, in turn, lovingly supported us with calls, emails,and constant postings on Facebook which I accessed on a tiny portable computer in my room. I confess to total wipe-out at the end of each day, but morning found me revived and ready to go again. When I brought him home, Tom required some specialized care, but I had expert and welcome help from home nurses and physical therapists during the period immediately following his discharge.

Now the patient is well on the way to full recovery and I, looking back on this suddenly imposed leap into deep water, am filled with intense gratitude and astonishment. I know now that I have regained my life. I judge my health to be 99+% regained, and I am continuing to work the DNRS program with a goal of no less than 100% health.

A true saying: "Never say never". Having experienced this rebirth, thanks to Annie Hopper, I have been given a new chance at a full life, and thanks to skilled surgeons and others, Tom has as well. I'd say the timing is nothing less than perfect, wouldn't you?

CHAPTER 17

At the End of Her Rope and Praying For a Miracle

Before she came to the program, Jessica had been suffering from a limbic system impairment for about eight years. For six of those years, she was completely disabled.

The cause of Jessica's limbic system impairment was a perfect storm of stressors. Within a one month period, she had Prednisone/Steroid poisoning and Benadryl toxicity from two prescribed over-doses, she had moved into a house with *Stachybotrys* (black) mould, and she had suffered a head injury from a car accident. Prior to this, Jessica had been hospitalized for a couple of months due to a virus, and she had had vaccine injuries from immunizations for international travel, recommended by her primary care physician.

With the help of an environmental doctor, Jessica was able to improve somewhat, but never really fully recovered from that lethal combination that caused trauma to her limbic system. She was managing to live, but was struggling from day to day.

After giving birth to her beautiful daughter, Jessica developed new conditions, including fibromyalgia, chronic pain, and chronic migraines. Giving birth was a miracle in itself as all of her doctors had told her that she would never be able to carry a baby to term, or if she did, that her baby would have endless health problems. Her baby was born perfectly healthy. But after giving birth, Jessica's condition quickly deteriorated, and she found herself at a point that was even worse than where she had started. The hormones from pregnancy and the stress of childbirth reactivated her limbic system trauma in a big way.

Jessica could not leave her house. She lives in a very hot climate in Southern California where temperatures routinely reach 115 degrees Fahrenheit/46 degrees Celsius. However, Jessica could not tolerate air conditioning or many heating systems because she had become sensitive to propylene glycol, which is used in heating and in air conditioning. This meant that she could not go into the majority of buildings. She could not be in an airconditioned car. She could not go to the grocery store, the doctor's office, the hospital, or most public places. She was trapped like a caged bird in her home – like one of the millions of other 'canaries' that are warning us of the toxins found in our daily environment.

Jessica was essentially disabled.

Like others with limbic system impairment, Jessica had spent years and thousands of dollars looking for answers. Jessica had been working as an actress in film and TV and, as a result, she had the means to pursue a number of options for healing. Over the years, she was diagnosed with the following conditions: unidentified auto-immune syndrome, postural orthostatic tachycardia syndrome, premature ventricular contractions, attention deficit hyperactivity disorder, mould biotoxin illness, extreme multiple chemical sensitivities, environmental illness, fibromyalgia, chronic fatigue syndrome, chronic pain syndrome, genetic detoxification inefficiency gene, chronic migraines, electric hypersensitivity syndrome, heavy metal toxicity and food sensitivities. She also experienced the associated depression, anxiety and obsessive-compulsive behaviours that often accompany these conditions.

In the first two years of her illness, Jessica spent $300,000 and over eight years, she spent a total of three quarters of a million dollars looking for an answer. Jessica lists the treatments that she tried:

> For several years, I did a complete environmental medicine protocol with bioidentical supplements and herbs to support my liver, kidneys, detoxification and immune functions, because it was believed that that was the issue. I did infrared sauna, exercised with oxygen, dieted, juiced, cleansed and flushed myself to the moon and back. I'm as clean as a whistle, so technically, if that theory were completely true, I'd be healed by now.
>
> I have been to the best specialists in the country, in the world. I was sent to the Mayo Clinic. I used to say "How many specialists does it take to screw in a light bulb," because none of them could figure it out. The top neurologist and the top endocrinologists couldn't figure it out. Most of them thought I was crazy, or that I was a guinea pig, and that they just had to keep testing me and they'd eventually find it. But they didn't.
>
> I've done everything. You name it, I've done it. Emotional Freedom Technique, tapping, craniosacral therapy, psychotherapy, colour therapy, aroma therapy, music therapy, sound healing, chanting mantras, yoga, physical therapy, Qi Gong, Martial Arts and Medical Qi Gong, acupuncture and traditional Chinese medicine, massage therapy, kinesiology/muscle testing, special diets, Sublingual Immunotherapy, Provocation/Neurtralization.... I mean, you name the spiritual path, physiological approach, technique or modality, I tried it — and I worked it to the bone.

Shamanic work, juicing, cleanses, fasting, heavy metal chelation, hydro colon therapy, frequency specific micro-current/electric treatments, personal work, life-coaching, copious amounts of belief work — all of it, including meditation, positive thinking and affirmations. And I bought enough supplements to fill the Empire State building. None of it worked. None of it.

When these things started happening, I thought I could heal myself. I am certified in many different healing modalities and have studied extensively with some of the world's greatest spiritual teachers and healers. For almost eight years, I believed I was doing everything physically possible to heal myself, and it didn't work. I went to see all the greatest healers in the world – all the sages and saints and swamis and masters and shamans – all of them. You name the spiritual path or technique or modality, I've tried it, and I've worked it deeply, passionately and thoroughly.

And what happened was — I took it personally. I took it personally that I could not heal myself. I took my limbic system injury personally, as if there were something fundamentally wrong with me or that I was cursed or being punished somehow. Maybe I didn't deserve to be healed, to be well. Maybe I was paying a price for something I had done in the past. Maybe this imprisonment and recurring terror, this seeming death-sentence was my fate, my destiny and I just had to accept it. I used to have such an amazing, full, incredible life, and felt smote by God, cast out of the garden. What had I done wrong?

This type of thinking resulted in critical self-talk, negative core beliefs, and truly harmful and self-sabotaging emotional behaviours, and a loss of belief in myself.

Jessica got to the point where she did not want to live anymore. She felt that she had tried "everything" and had given up hope. She recounts:

> I came to my fiance one night and I said, "I'm done. I want to die. That's it. I can't do it anymore. I can't be a partner to you, I can't be a mother to my daughter. I'm not living life. I'm not even existing. I'm not even just surviving instead of thriving. I'm a walking dead person. This isn't life. This isn't who I am."
>
> I went outside and lay down at the feet of a statue of Mother Mary that I have in my backyard. I lay there and cried, begged and prayed for some kind of miracle. I simply could not take it anymore.
>
> Meanwhile, my partner started searching YouTube and he typed in 'cure for multiple chemical sensitivities.' The next morning, he said, "Honey, check your inbox, the title says 'cure for multiple chemical sensitivities.' And I said, "Yeah, I checked my email and I saw that BS!" I was like, "Yeah, cure for MCS — yeah, right."
>
> It took me two weeks to open the email. Every day, my partner would say, "Have you looked at that email? Honey, why don't you open that email?" So two weeks later, I finally moved past my resistance, and I watched the testimony of Bil. And it was like a miracle — but I wouldn't let myself feel it all the way.
>
> So I watched the next testimonial, the photographer who did the NY Times piece [Thilde Jensen]. And I was like — there's something to this. And then I went to the DNRS website link. And I saw Annie Hopper's face, and I saw her sparkling eyes, and I started crying because I knew I'd found it — and my body said, "Yes! Yes! Yes!" And then

stunned, I watched Tyffanee's video because I had also suf-
fered from anaphylactic reactions for six years. When I
heard Tyffanee's story, I cried and cried because I knew if
Tyffanee could do it — I could do it. I knew that the Divine
Mother had been listening, and when I looked and saw
Annie's shining face, I knew there was a way out.

Jessica attended the live program that we held in her home-town in January, 2014. Jessica had some huge "A-Ha" moments during the program. However, her new understandings were only the beginning of her recovery process. She describes them in the following:

Psychologically, I have had some huge realizations,
really big light bulbs coming up. When I came in, I thought
I had all these different conditions: these seemingly dis-
parate things – from chronic fatigue syndrome, fibromy-
algia, multiple chemical sensitivities, postural orthostatic
tachycardia syndrome, electric hypersensitivity syndrome,
chronic migraines, pain, obsessive compulsive disorders,
depression, food sensitivities, attention deficit disorder, etc.
I was told that I had all these illnesses. And that used to
overwhelm me, and I realized that was also a chronic pat-
tern – being overwhelmed. Throughout the course, I real-
ized these were all originating from the same dysfunction,
they were part of a greater whole and by addressing the
root, all of the different symptoms and conditions started
to shift because it's a singular origin with many branches.
I have noticed my sense of smell shifted – where I used
to smell something and be afraid of it, I now enjoy it, or I
simply notice it and I smell it, but there's no panic or fear
or anxiety. There's calm. My system stays calm. So, I still

have the sense of smell, but I don't have all those unhealthy things that follow that. That's a huge victory for me.

I've noticed that pain has decreased and sometimes I forget pain exists. I am sleeping like a baby, all the way through the night. I am waking up happy and energized and refreshed. It's almost foreign to me for the alarm to go off and for me to sit up in bed and be ready to go for my day. My vision has changed. I can focus. It's like getting to experience the world through new eyes. And some of the changes, ironically, don't feel like changes in the sense that I feel more like I've reclaimed myself. The me I used to be is coming back! And that is electric – that feeling of reclaiming myself and my personality, my emotions, my outlook on life, my joy, my optimism. Who I really am.

On an emotional level — I'm happy! And I haven't been able to say I'm happy in so many years.

Realizing that I had a brain injury has helped me to understand all of the things I had been experiencing that seemed like a mystery. There's a legitimate injury in the brain that has to be addressed. It has to be addressed in a literal, physiological way and with knowledge of neuro-plasticity-based techniques to harness the brain's ability to go back into itself and rewire itself.

So I would say: Don't take it personally if everything that you have tried hasn't worked. It truly is not personal. It is neurological, it is an injury, and it is not your "fault."

If what you have tried doesn't work, it's because it is not dealing with the root of the illness. This is about a brain injury. This is a limbic system dysfunction. And it takes an in-depth, experiential knowledge of neuroscience and neuroplasticity to be able to undo the ball of yarn that got wrapped up in the first place by the injury. It is not *something we can think our way out of. It's not just about positive affirmations, changing some core beliefs, positive self-talk, etc. We must first be educated as to how the brain works, and how it is able to change itself. Then, we must learn and develop the neuroplasticity-based tools and skills to be able to work with the brain, to speak with it in its own language.*

It is like the mechanics of a car. I understand how an engine works. I have a basic understanding of cars. I know what the fuel filter is and how the carburetor works. But if you ask me to replace the engine, I wouldn't be able to — because I'm not a mechanic! Annie is like the expert, head auto mechanic. She studied, developed, and implemented these techniques. She knows how to help you go into the engine, flush, rewire and replace the parts, in order to thoroughly and completely heal this injury.

Limbic system dysfunction needs to be addressed on all levels, and the core level is the brain itself. Basically, what Annie does is teach us how to be mechanics and repair our own brains. Once you come to the course or do the DVDs, it's very liberating – because then you understand, whereas before it was a mystery. It was like I was trying to be a mechanic, yet I didn't know how to replace a car engine, but now I'm being given the tools.

I had an epiphany. Not being able to heal myself wasn't about my spiritual aptitude or my level of consciousness or my skills as a healer — it was simply that I didn't know the techniques. I didn't know the neuroscience behind what it takes to heal the brain from limbic system injury.

So don't take yourself personally. Don't take your brain injury personally. Don't take the fact all of your previous efforts or your spiritual practice didn't heal you, person-

ally. Just come to the course and you'll be given the tools. Then you will truly be able to step into yourself, into your power and heal your brain through legitimate, cutting-edge neuroscience.

What we learn in this program is that, yes, chemicals can be harmful, certain levels of them can be toxic and can create injuries. They aren't always the best things for the oceans, the forests, the animals, or people, but reacting to them in a way that is completely debilitating and disabling is not normal. A neurotypical person does not have a seemingly life-threatening response to minute amount of chemicals. This is an indicator that there is an injury in the brain and that the limbic system is in a state of imbalance.

What the program is saying is that, yes, we want to care for the earth. Yes, we want to honour and respect humanity, the earth and all of life on this planet. We want to be environmentally conscious because it's the right thing to do. The program is not ignoring that. The program is about rewiring our brains to a healthy place so we can interact with the world in a positive, calm, relaxed and freeing, expansive, enjoyable way. It is about transforming our health and reclaiming our lives so that we can be of service to humanity and the earth from a place of joy, health and well-being, from a place of ease and happiness, from a place of celebration.

Being part of a group in this work was incredible. Nothing can compare to it because there is a tangible, kinetic energy in the recovery process where, as you witness other people recovering, you also feel and experience your own recovery through observing them. As they grow, shift and change, you realize that you are doing the same. There are days when you have challenges or valleys, and it's everything you can do to just muster your way through, and then someone in the group shares, and they speak your heart, and you realize you're not alone, and their hope gives you hope. Even if you don't feel it at that moment, you see the palpable recovery in someone else, and you know that if they can do it, you can do it.

Doing the program with a group is so empowering because as you see each person heal and shift, you can feel yourself heal and shift. Every victory you see in another member of the group is your victory. Their joy is your joy; you're doing it together. You're holding space for one another, you're encouraging and celebrating one another. And sometimes the group holds you up. You are not alone, and just this human connection in and of itself — when life used to be so isolated — is deeply healing.

If you can get to an in-person program, the connections that are made in these groups are magical, profound and lasting. They are soul connections, they are heart connections, they are mind connections. There's a special healing, a faith, and a hope that is truly medicine for the heart and the soul.

We know scientifically that the brain can heal itself, and I have had this legitimate, physical experience. I have watched my brain change itself, and then I have watched different symptoms change and morph and disappear right in front of my eyes. I've seen it happen to the whole group.

The writing is on the wall; neuroplasticity is real, neuroplasticity therapy works. It's saving lives, it's saving my life. There is so much hope.

When I asked Jessica what she would say to someone who is still suffering, she replied:

I would say to anyone who's suffering from limbic system impairment:

Don't give up. There is a way out, and you can do it. It is not too late, it is never too late. There is hope for you and you CAN get your life back — I am living proof! Just hang on, keep putting one foot in front of the other and do whatever it takes to get to DNRS. Take this program. Take it! Take it! Take it! If you can't make it in person at first, order the DVDs and use that last bit of energy you've got to do the program. Commit fully and you will go all the way! Don't let go of the rope, keep going. All you need to do is get this information and get the tools. Once you have the tools, you will realize that they are a ladder up and out of the abyss. Take this program – you can and WILL reclaim your life, as I have. It will give you your life back. It will give you yourself back. This is more precious than gold! And you are worth it. To come out of the darkness and into the light of life again, to freely live and delight in the world again, brimming with energy and vibrant health — is a miracle and a magnificent joy, beyond words.

The following is something Jessica wrote on the members-only community forum, five months after attending the live program:

Hello Dynamos! I just want to express my deep GRATITUDE for this AMAZING program and recovery process. It truly is a miraculous practice and process that has gifted me a life, MY LIFE, back--indeed given me a whole NEW life, that I couldn't believe was possible, a few months ago.

This morning I woke up early with M, made breakfast, dropped the dogs at the groomer's and chatted with the owner, as a huge, perfumed Poodle was being trimmed. I drove through freshly "hot topped"/paved roads all over town--with the windows down, I went to a large estate where the maids were cleaning with chemical-based cleaners and WOW. NO SYMPTOMS, and not even a thought of symptoms. Was in there for 15 min, chatting away by the laundry room where they were using traditional soap and fabric softener sheets. I was happy as a clam, and clear as a bell. Didn't even register it on my radar. Wasn't until I left that I realized how awesome that was. Then I went to the local market to pick up some items for lunch, chatted up the folks there, laughing, grinning, beaming and appreciating every SECOND of the experience, even walking through the aisle with traditional cleaning/laundry products. I am TOO HAPPY to let any of that affect me, bounces right off me, because NOTHING can take away my recovery, my deep value for the present moment which I cherish with the very CORE of my being--because 5 months ago I couldn't even WALK THROUGH this store and now here I am, bursting with JOY and owning the place. And I LOVE being able to go anywhere I want with ease and grace, I TREASURE being able to do simple things like purchase groceries for my family to prepare food and enliven my home with fresh, healthy, home-cooked delights. On my gas stove. 3 times per day. Heck YEAH! I LOVE THIS LIFE.

Then for the fun of it, I decided to go to my awesome, happy, luminous chiropractor and get a sweet little adjustment. Why? Because 5 months ago I couldn't do this because she used air conditioning and now I CAN DO ANYTHING. And I like to FEEL GOOD. And she told me that for the first time since she'd met me, that I was "...presenting with a completely normal nervous system. Congratulations." Why, of course I am!

And as I coasted home, all happy and relaxed, singing and listening to some beautiful Indian chanting music "Shri Ram, Jai Ram" (which means Great Creator, Victorious Creator), savoring and appreciating the sweet, cool AC blowing against my face on this very hot day, ogling the gorgeous mighty mountains at the head of my street--it struck me. Just how very, very NORMAL I was. How very normal I AM. And that 5 months ago, I couldn't have done ANY of these things that I just did today with effortless ease, calm, peace, grace and JOY. Like it was nothing. And in that moment it was EVERYTHING. And I fully comprehended in every cell the MIRACLE that has become my life. The Miracle of this work. This MIRACLE that Annie has created and gifted to us, so that we may create and live our own miracles. And the tears rolled and washed over me like a mighty ocean. That this is REAL.

THANK YOU, Annie. Thank you so very much. And Thank You Great, Victorious Creator, for my life. And Thank Me for loving myself enough to Create a Miracle, through my commitment to this revolutionary practice.

Jessica was a guest speaker at one of the DNRS programs four months after taking the program herself.

I'm a regular person now. I have recovered from things that I was told were impossible to recover from.... I'm further along in four months [of DNRS] than I was in three years of an environmental medical protocol. I know it's because I'm addressing the root, I'm not approaching it from the symptoms – I'm approaching it from the origin — which is a brain injury.

While addressing the class, she spoke about her spiritual mentor of many years. When people were really suffering, they would say to him, "I have no reason to have faith, I have no evidence or proof of anything to give me faith that my life can change. How am I supposed to have faith?"

He would respond, "Faith is the belief in the experience of others. If your faith in yourself is challenged, you can hear and see and know the experience of others. If it is possible for them, it is possible for you."

CHAPTER 18

My Doctor Thought that I had Multiple Sclerosis

For five long and tortuous years, Paula had suffered from anxiety, depression and post traumatic stress disorder. The symptoms of depression started soon after her sons were born. But Paula did not tell anyone how she was feeling. She hid her feelings like a dirty secret. Often she felt shame for feeling the way that she did. After all, shouldn't she be happy? She had two healthy boys and really had nothing to complain about. Life was good – or so it seemed from the outside looking in. But inside, Paula felt as if she was dying a very slow and painful death.

Paula hit her "tipping point" after a foot surgery where she chose to have surgery while still awake. She was not in a healthy place emotionally before the surgery and felt pushed by her surgeon to go through with it. She opted not to have anesthetic as she thought that her recovery time would be less without it. This deadly combination of depression, anxiety and fear with the surgery created the perfect recipe for disaster. The day after the surgery she started having panic attacks and full-blown posttraumatic stress disorder. She was constantly in a state of 'fight-or-flight'.

Paula felt as if she was slowly being squeezed out of everything in her life. She had gone to the doctor with her concerns, but her doctor just placed her in a "generalized anxiety" category.

Paula had become fearful all of the time, and she couldn't control it, and she certainly didn't want to talk about it.

Then the bizarre physical symptoms started to happen. Things that she couldn't explain. Constant pain and aching in her neck and shoulders, headaches, numbness and tingling, loss of balance, feeling overwhelmed by the smallest of sounds. Everything in her environment was becoming a perceived threat.

As the illness continued to progress, Paula went back to her doctor. Paula was not prepared for what her doctor told her during one of her visits.

Paula recalls the moment:

> *I remember that day very clearly. I was in her office and she told me 'Paula, this can be MS.' I was really discouraged at that time because I really tried to help myself through this process. I didn't go to the doctor expecting to hear those words. The worst part is that there was nothing that they could do for me. I felt very discouraged and helpless. It was like a waiting game to see how long it took me to completely fall apart.*

When Paula was at her worst, her visual and auditory processing were extremely heightened. Even the smallest sounds like a ticking clock or the sound of an appliance would trigger a panic attack. It felt uncontrollable. Paula describes what it was like to try to go grocery shopping:

> *If I would walk into a store, like a grocery store, the overhead fans or lights and noises and just that vast space of those stores was too much and I couldn't handle it. I*

wanted to hit the ground because I had no sense of balance. I would have to hold on to the shelves when I was walking. I just was thrown off completely and I couldn't control it.

Paula would often awake in the middle of the night in a panic attack. As the list of symptoms continued to worsen, she also developed sensitivity to electro magnetic fields. Paula didn't even realize that there was such a thing. But with sharing her symptoms with a couple of people, she discovered that what she was feeling was real. Eventually Paula had to quit her job due to the illness.

Paula describes what life was like:

So basically, bottom line, I was depressed and I was disconnected from life. I was totally, 100% on the path of illness and if it wasn't for this program, I would have died a slow death. And my children would not have the mom that they have today.

Paula saw a number of different health care professionals during this time, searching for relief and answers. She saw an MS doctor, specialists, physiotherapists, chiropractors, massage therapists, naturopathic doctors and reiki masters to name a few. And while some of them were valuable, and some are still part of her team today, they did not offer her the help that she needed.

Paula describes it like this:

From all the treatment that I've utilized you can easily come to the conclusion that it was a lot of money. Thousands of dollars were spent on me trying to get well. The number would still be adding up today if it wasn't for this program. It stopped the financial bleed 100%. And really, it's the best dollars I've ever invested. It's given me the greatest return and you can't put a price on your health. Without it you really do have nothing.

Feeling desperate and hopeless one night, Paula decided to share her feelings and her bizarre list of physical symptoms with her friend. Her friend Teresa listened patiently as Paula described the nightmare that had become her life. When Paula finished, Teresa said, "I used to know a woman who suffered from a lot of the same things that you are describing. Let me see if I still have her contact information." Serendipitously, I was the person that Teresa was referring to. Teresa and I had lost touch years ago and she knew that I had gotten sick but didn't know what had happened to me. I was no longer on her contact list so she "googled" the name Annie Hopper and voila, my website popped up.

Paula immediately signed up for the next program and well, the rest is history. She realized that healing the limbic system is an inside job; no one else can do it for you.

Paula goes on to say:

> *Annie gives us the tools and the strategies to help heal our limbic systems from trauma. And when this underlying cause is addressed the rest just falls into place naturally. It's nothing short of a miracle.*

Paula was very disciplined with implementing the program on a daily basis. She fully realized that rewiring her limbic system would take both motivation and a daily commitment.

Paula describes the changes that she had noticed:

The changes that I have experienced since taking this program and committing to daily practice have been beyond amazing and beyond anything I could have ever imagined.

I felt a shift immediately during the program and that just gave me the momentum and the desire to want to commit to this. The daily positive changes that kept happening kept me focused and kept me on track. I felt more awake than I had ever felt and my mental fog was lifted. I could hear the whispers of my heart – like my soul was coming alive. I was no longer living with all these negative thoughts in my head. Then my body was responding physically. It was amazing. And I was no longer living in fear; I was like this kid. It felt like my eyes were wide open and everything that I was seeing was like the first time. I went into this program with the hopes of physically healing and the mental and emotional healing that occurred was the greatest side effect ever. The freedom I feel to this day is beyond amazing. My soul has been set free and I'm no longer held back by my limitations and my limbic system is running on a new program. I am available for all opportunities that come my way. I was followed at the MS clinic for 4 years and just this last August I was cleared and given the green light. So thankfully, that door is closed and that is behind me as well.

In fact, Paula was surprised because she had forgotten what it was like when she was living with illness two years ago.

It's so incredible that we can actually forget the pain that we were in when it's gone.

When I asked Paula what she would say to someone who is still suffering, she replied:

> Firstly, have faith in your ability to do this. You hold the power to heal your body. This program will give you the tools necessary to retrain your brain for lasting success. If your brain can change for the worse, it can change for the better. This I know. I have also come to realize how we can read all the books out there and they all tell us we can have this wonderful life. We know when we read it that it makes sense, but they don't show us how to achieve this. The Dynamic Neural Retraining System bridges that gap. It gives you a system and a protocol that's going take you from suffering to thriving. The program shows you how to get there.
>
> You just have to be brave and you just have to trust in this process and take the first step. I have come to learn that whatever you need in life will be given to you. I even tell myself, Paula, you know, why do you even worry? When are you gonna get it? Whatever you're worried about either isn't going to happen or seriously, if it does, then somebody shows up or something shows up and guess what, you're able to deal with it, it's that easy. That's the beauty of life. So I just say stop trying to figure it out. Just show up in life and be present and you'll know what to do and how to do it.

Paula has also applied the program to other areas of her life since recovering from limbic system dysfunction.

When she had recovered, she suffered from a concussion that she got while playing hockey. The night after the concussion she woke up in the middle of the night in a panic attack. That hadn't happened since she attended the program. Paula recognized that her brain was going back into a trauma pattern. Paula immediately contacted one of our DNRS Coaches who assured her that she could use the program to assist her in preventing her brain from going down that trauma pattern again. Paula started to practice again and feels confident that applying the program after the concussion helped in her recovery process.

Paula also mentioned how she became emotionally available to other people in her life. Paula goes on to say:

> I am available to help my brother in his journey to heal from a reoccurring brain tumor. I wouldn't have been able to be there for him if I hadn't healed with the program. It's amazing that this time that should be full of fear and worry and anxiety and sadness has actually been some of the greatest highs and moments of joy that I've ever felt. And that's the hugest paradox ever.
>
> I will never go back into those darkest days of depression no matter what. Yeah, we're human and I can still experience sadness and hurt and fear but just like Annie says, you're the observer, I see them for what they are and I learn. You move on – you move through it. It's hard to fathom but it's beyond amazing. I feel so blessed. So yes, my life has been nothing but a miracle since that day. I appreciate every day and moment. My children have this mother that's alive and living. And my heart is just full of love and gratitude. You are all worthy of this same feeling.
>
> Basically what I've learned from all of this is that we can only heal as a team. While it's true that each of us has to do the work and have the desire, we need to be supported by others on the way. This program is amazing because it gives you support. When I reached out they were there. So it's awesome. Annie had to first do the work on herself and

build her story and gain support and look at how many people she is able to reach and help because of that. And by her helping me, I can now go on and be available to those that need me and be inspiring in life to others. It's just this huge ripple affect.

It's hard to believe how many things I've done in only 2 years. It kind of defies logic. Time isn't linear to me anymore, and my energy is no longer proportional to how many hours of sleep I get each night. It's just like this untapped potential inside of me that's there when I need it. And when you live from a place of passion and purpose and you're plugged in, well, you just can't stop me.

When Paula came to speak at an information night for the program she ended her talk with the following quote from the book *The Alchemist (by Paulo Coelho, Editorio Rocco Ltd., 1988)*. The quote came to her when she was taking the progam. To this day, Paula still has the quote posted on her wall. It says:

Decisions are only the beginning of something. When someone makes a decision, he is, in fact, plunging into a powerful current that carries him to a place he had never even dreamed of when he made that initial decision.

Thank you Paula for making the decision to take the program. For making the decision that you are worth the work that it takes to create your own miracle, and for making the decision to share your inspiring story with others. Your recovery will touch the hearts of many and give them the hope and the courage that they need to be a part of the ripple effect.

CHAPTER 19

Global Implications for Self-Directed Neuroplasticity

The power to change our brain structure and function through our own free will is remarkable, and perhaps even more than this, it is empowering. The application of this knowledge has the ability to transform millions of lives. Far from merely being victims of illness, when armed with the right knowledge and tools, we can effectively tap into our own self-healing abilities.

We are now realizing that diseases we thought were intractable in the past are now effectively being treated through self-directed neuroplasticity. Not only does this discovery and understanding have the potential to help millions of people in their recovery process, this new application of neuroplasticity has the potential to revolutionize the field of health care. We are just scratching the surface in our understanding of the potential of the human brain and its role in overall health and the healing process. Indeed, this is truly an exciting time for the field of psychoneuroimmunology and the vast implications in this area are monumental. Yet more research needs to be done to validate the transformations in health that are taking place and we are actively seeking collaboration in this area.

However, as exciting as this breakthrough is, I temper my excitement about the future with the fact that many common illnesses that people suffer from are directly related to limbic system dysfunction and a maladapted stress response that is, in part, activated by the toxic environment that we live in. With this in mind, our focus also needs to be on prevention of illness, not just treatment of illness.

I cannot help but think of the millions who are yet to become sick – unless there is massive change in the way that we live on the planet. As a society, we have naively introduced chemicals and new technology into our daily lives without knowing – or bothering to adequately research and understand – the consequences. So many of the illnesses that I've written about in this book have only been in existence since the Second World War. It would be naïve to think that, as a species, we would be unaffected by the environment that we've created. On a very fundamental level, I recognize that what is happening to the planet is also happening to humanity on a global level. With this in mind I would highly recommend that you become proactive in your awareness about how your environment may be affecting your health and take active steps to help create a healthy home and workplace. There are many resources to help you in this regard. For example, the Environmental Working Group (EWG) has a large database of information. EWG empowers people to live healthier lives in a healthier environment. Their website address is www.ewg.org.

I also realize that limbic system rehabilitation does not replace common sense. Developing a high degree of environmental awareness, eating nutritious food, regular exercise, establishing balance in our lives, strengthening our social connections and managing stress are essential in order to maintain and promote good health.

For those who are suffering from limbic system impairment, my heart goes out to you. Please do not lose hope. There is an answer, and there is a way to regain your health.

Navigating limbic system trauma can be challenging and is best addressed with supervision. Limbic system trauma alters one's ability to think, to be objective, and to feel safe in the world. It alters the brain's normal filtering process, which increases its vulnerability and keeps it in a cycle of trauma. To truly grasp that recovery is possible, one needs to embrace the idea that brain function plays a key role in optimal health. This does not mean that the illness is 'all in your head,' but rather that recovery, through neuroplasticity, requires that the brain be involved in the rehabilitation process.

Keep in mind that the DNRS program and limbic system rehabilitation is experiential and accumulative in nature. With repetition, the new neural patterns will make themselves apparent, and symptoms of illness will decrease. From that moment forward, the physical, emotional, and psychological changes will provide evidence of recovery.

Self-directed neuroplasticity represents a new paradigm in treating chronic and mysterious illnesses. Just like the people featured in this book, you have the power to wire your brain for healing, transform your health, and reclaim your life!

Be well and make healthy choices!

With sincere love and gratitude,

Annie

Works Cited

A

Antoni, M.H., Lutgendorf, S.K., Blomberg, B., Carver, C.S., Lechner, S., Diaz, A., Stagl, J., Arevalo, J.M., & Cole, S.W. (2012). Cognitive-behavioral stress management reverses anxiety-related leukocyte transcriptional dynamics. *Biological Psychiatry 71(4)*, 366-372.

Armour, J. A. (2007). The little brain on the heart. *Cleveland Clinic Journal of Medicine, Volume 74, Supplement 1.* http://www.ccjm.org/content/74/Suppl_1/S48.full.pdf+html?sid=cdd08633-ac07-45b0-be76-9266120337eb

Ashirmetov, A.K. & Krakovskiĭ, M.E. (1990). The role of the parasympathetic nervous system in the regulation of microsomal monooxygenase activity in the liver of rats. *Fiziologicheskiĭ Zhurnal, 36(6)*, 43-46.

B

Bolte Taylor, J., (2006). *My Stroke of Insight*, Viking.

Brown, R.P., & Gerbarg, P. L. (2005). Sudarshan Kriya Yogic Breathing in the Treatment of Stress, Anxiety, and Depression: Part 1 – Neurophysiologic Model. *The Journal of Alternative and Complementary Medicine, 11(1)*, 189-201.

C

Clodi, M., Vila, G., Geyeregger, R., Riedl, M., Stulnig, T. M., Struck, J., Luger, T.A., & Luger, A. (2008). Oxytocin alleviates the neuroendocrine and cytokine response to bacterial endotoxin in healthy men. *American Journal of Physiology – Endocrinology and Metabolism 295*, E686-E691.

Cohen, S., Janicki-Deverts D., Doyle, W.J., Miller, G.E., Frank, E., Rabin, B.S., & Turner, R. (2012). Chronic stress, glucocorticoid receptor resistance, inflammation, and disease risk. *Proceedings of National Academy of Sciences of the United States, 109(16),* 5995-5999. http://www.pnas.org/content/109/16/5995.full.pdf17.

Cole, S. W., Hawkley, L. C., Arevalo, J. M., Sung, C. Y., Rose, R. M., & Cacioppo, J. T. (2007). Social regulation of gene expression in human leukocytes. *Genome Biology 8(9),* R189.

Creswell J.D., Irwin M.R., Burklund L.J., Lieberman M.D., Arevalo J.M., Ma, J., Breen E.C., & Cole S.W. (2012). Mindfulness-based stress reduction training reduces loneliness and pro-inflammatory gene expression in older adults: a small randomized controlled trial. *Brain, Behavior, and Immunity 2(7),* 1095-1101.

D

Dispenza, J. (2007). *Evolve Your Brain.* Health Communications, Inc.

Dispenza, J. (2012). *Breaking the Habit of Being Yourself.* Hay House.

Doidge, N. (2007). *The Brain That Changes Itself.* Viking Penguin.

F

Friedman, A., Kaufer, D., Shemer J., Hendler, I., Soreq, H., & Tur-Kaspa I. (1996). Pyridostigmine brain penetration under stress enhances neuronal excitability and induces early immediate transcriptional response. *Nature Medicine 2,* 1382-1385.

G

Gershon, M.D., Welch, M.G., Anwar, M., Chang, C.Y., Gross, K.J., & Ruggiero, D.A. (2010). Combined administration of secretin and oxytocin inhibits chronic colitis and associated activation of forebrain neurons. *Neurogastroenterology and Motility 22(6),* 654-e202.

Gilbert, B. (2010). The neurobiology of anxiety: perception of danger runs deep.*Parkhurst Exchange,* 18(02). www.parkhurstexchange.com/columns/psychiatry/feb10_anxiety.

Goleman, D. (1996). *Emotional Intelligence: Why It Can Matter More Than IQ.* Bloomsbury Publishing.

H

Haley, R. (2008). *Gulf War Syndrome and Brain Damage.* UT Southwestern.

Hebb, D. (1949). *The Organization of Behavior.* Wiley and Sons.

Hermans, E. J., *et al.* (2011). Stress-Related Noradrenergic Activity Prompts Large-Scale Neural Network Reconfiguration. *American Association for the Advancement of Science 334,1151-1153.*

Hillert, L., Jovanovic, H., Ahs, F., & Savic, I. (2013). Women with Multiple Chemical Sensitivity Have Increased Harm Avoidance and Reduced 5-HT(1A) Receptor Binding Potential in the Anterior Cingulate and Amygdala. *PLoS ONE, 8(1):e54781.*

Hillert, L., Musabasic, D., Berglund, H., Ciumas, C., & Savic, I. (2007). Odor processing in multiple chemical sensitivity. *Human Brain Mapping, 28(3),* 172-182.

Holzschneider, K. & C. Mulert. (2011). Neuroimaging in anxiety disorders. *Dialogues in Clinical Neuroscience, 13(4),* 453–461. http://www.ncbi.nlm.nih.gov/pmc/articles/PMC3263392/#!po=3.33333.

Hopper, A. (2012). Emotional Rescue. *Kelowna Capital News. April 9, 2011, June 5, 2011, Feb.16, 2013*

J

Jackson Nakazawa, D. (2013). *The Last Best Cure: My quest to awaken the healing parts of my brain and get back my body, my joy, and my life.* Hudson Street Press.

K

Katerndahl, D. A., Bell, I. R., Palmer, R. F., and Miller, C. S. (2012) Chemical intolerance in primary care settings: prevalence, comorbidity, and outcomes. *Annals of Family Medicine* (10:298-299).

Keller, A., Litzelman, K., Wisk, L.E., Maddox, T., Cheng, E.R., Creswell, P.D., & Witt, W.P. (2012). Does the perception that stress affects health matter? *Health Psychology, 31(5)*, 677-684.

Kiecolt-Glaser, J. K., Speicher, C. E., Holliday, J. E., & Glaser, R. (1984). Stress and the transformation of lymphocytes by Epstein-Barr virus. *Journal of Behavioral Medicine 7(1)*, 1-12.

Krukoff, T.L. & Khalili, P. (1997). Stress-induced activation of nitric oxide-producing neurons in the rat brain. *Journal of Comparative Neurology, 377(4)*, 509-19.

Krusemark, E.A., & Li, W. (2012). Enhanced olfactory sensory perception of threat in znxiety: zn event-related fMRI study. *Chemosensory Perception 5(1)*, 37-45.

L

Ledoux, J. E. (1996). *The Emotional Brain: The Mysterious Underpinnings of Emotional Life*. Simon & Schuster Paperbacks.

Lipton, B. H. (2005). *The Biology of Belief*. Hay House.

M

Mahmutyazicioglu, K., Konuk, N., Atasoy, N., Atik, L., & Gundogdu S. (2005). Evaluation of the hippocampus and the anterior cingulate gyrus by proton MR spectroscopy in patients with posttraumatic stress disorder. *Diagnostic and Interventional Radiology 11(3)*, 125-129.

McCraty, R. & Atkinson, M. (1999). Influence of afferent cardiovascular input on cognitive performance and alpha activity. *Proceedings of the Annual Meeting of the Pavlovian Society.*

McRae, K., Hughes, B., Chopra, S., Gabrieli, J.D., Gross, J. J., & Ochsner, K. N. (2010). The neural bases of distraction and reappraisal. *Journal of Cognitive Neuroscience, 22(2)*, 248-262.

Merchant, J. (2013). Immunology: the pursuit of happiness. *Nature: International Weekly Journal of Science, 503(7477)*. *http://www. nature.com/news/immunology-the-pursuit-of-happiness-1.14225.*

Miller, C. S., (1997). Toxicant-induced loss of tolerance – an emerging theory of disease? *Environmental Health Perspective, 105 Supplement 2: 445-53.*

Modinos, G., Ormel, J., & Aleman, A. (2010). Individual differences in dispositional mindfulness and brain activity involved in reappraisal of emotion. *Social Cognitive and Affective Neuroscience, 5(4),* 369–377.

N

Neimark, Jill. (2013). Extreme chemical sensitivity makes sufferers allergic to life. *Discover Magazine. http://discovermagazine. com/2013/nov/13-allergic-life.*

O

Oosthuizen, F., Wegener, G., & Harvey, B. H. (2005). Nitric oxide as inflammatory mediator in post-traumatic stress disorder (PTSD): Evidence from an animal model. *Neuropsychiatric Disease and Treatment, 1(2),* 109–123.

Orriols, R., Costa, R., Jacas, G., Castell, J., & Sunyer, J. (2009). Brain Dysfunction in Multiple Chemical Sensitivity. *Journal of the Neurological Science, 287(1-2),* 72– 78.

P

Pall, M. (2007). *Unexplained Illnesses: Disease Paradigm for Chronic Fatigue Syndrome, Multiple Chemical Sensitivity, Fibromyalgia, Post-Traumatic Stress Disorder, and Gulf War Syndrome.* Haworth Press, Inc.

Pavlov, V.A. & Tracey, K.J. (2005). The cholinergic anti-inflammatory pathway. *Brain, Behavior, Immunity, 19(6),* 493-499

Perreau-Linck E., Beauregard M., Gravel P., Paquette V., Soucy, J.P., Diksic, M., & Benkelfat, C. (2007). In vivo measurements of brain trapping of C-labelled alpha-methyl-L-tryptophan during acute changes in mood states. *Journal of Psychiatry and Neuroscience 32(6),* 430-434.

Pert, C. (1997). *Molecules of Emotion: Why You Feel The Way You Feel.* Scribner.

Pray, L. A. (2004). Epigenetics: genome, meet your environment. *The Scientist,*14-20.

R

Rauch, S. L., Shin, L.M., & Wright, C. (2003). Neuroimaging studies of amygdala function in anxiety disorders. *Annals of New York Academy of Science, 984,* 389-410.

Reik, W. & Walter, J. (2001). Genomic imprinting: parental influence on the genome. *Nature Reviews. Genetics 2(1),* 21-32.

S

Schwartz, J. & Beyette, B. (1997) *Brain lock: Free Yourself from Obsessive-Compulsive Behavior: A Four-Step Self-Treatment Method to Change Your Brain Chemistry.* Regan Books.

Shin, L.M., Rauch, S.L., & Pitman, R.K. (2006). Amygdala, medial prefrontal cortex, and hippocampal function in PTSD. *Annals of the New York Academy of Sciences 1071,* 67-79.

Shum F.W., Wu L.J., Zhao M.G., Toyoda H., Xu H., Ren M., Pinaud R., Ko S.W., Lee Y.S., Kaang B.K., & Zhuo M. (2007). Alteration of cingulate long-term plasticity and behavioral sensitization to inflammation by environmental enrichment. *Learning and Memory* 14(4), 304-12. http://www.ncbi.nlm.nih.gov/pmc/articles/PMC2216536/.

Shurick, A. A., Hamilton, J. R., Harris, L. T., Roy, A. K., Gross, J. J., & Phelps, E. A. (2012). Durable effects of cognitive restructuring on conditioned fear. *Emotion, 12(6),* 1393-1397.

Singer, R. & Johnson, D.D. *Recognizing neurotoxicity.* www.neurotox.com/documents/Recognizing_Neurotoxicity.doc.

Sloan, R. P., et al. (2007). RR interval variability is inversely related to inflammatory markers: the CARDIA study. *Molecular Medicine, 13(3-4),* 178-184.

WIRED FOR HEALING

Statistics Canada, (2010). *The Canadian Community Health Survey (CCHS)*. Government of Canada.

Surani, M. A. (2001). Reprogramming of genome function through epigenetic inheritance. *Nature 414,* 122-128

V
_____

Vincent, S.R. & Kimura, H. (1992). Histochemical mapping of nitric oxide synthase in the rat brain. *Neuroscience, 46(4),* 755–784.

Volk, Steve. (2013). Rewiring the brain to treat OCD. *Discover Magazine. http://discovermagazine.com/2013/nov/14-defense-free-will.*

W
_____

Watkins, L.R., & Maier, S.F. (1999). Implications of immune-to-brain communication for sickness and pain. *Proceedings of the National Academy of Sciences of the United States of America, 96(14),* 7710-7713.

Wikipedia. http://en.wikipedia.org/wiki/Amygdala_hijack.

Wyller, V.B. (2007). The chronic fatigue syndrome--an update. *Acta neurologica Scandinavica. Supplementum 187,* 7–14.

APPENDIX A

Books and Articles of Note

A

Amen, D. G. (1998) *Change Your Brain; Change Your Life.* Three Rivers Press.

B

Begley, S. (2007). *Train Your Mind, Change Your Brain.* Ballantine Books.

Bolte Taylor, J. (1999) *My Stroke of Insight.* Viking Penguin.

D

De Raedt, R. (2006). Does neuroscience hold promise for further development of behaviour therapy? The case of emotional change after exposure in anxiety and depression. *Scandinavian Journal of Psychology, 47(3),* 225-36.

E

Emmer, B. J., et al. (2006). Damage to amygdala might cause neuropsychiatric symptoms in patients with systemic lupus erythematosus. *PubMed.gov Dec 3(12),* e499.

H

Hooper, M. (2003) *Engaging with Multiple Chemical Sensitivity (MCS).* Sunderland University, London.

K

Kensinger, E. and Corkin, S. (2004) Two routes to emotional memory: distinct neural processes for valence and arousal. *Proceedings of the National Academy of Sciences of the United States of America, 101(9)*, 3310–3315.

L

Landgrebe, M., Barta, W., Rosengarth, K., Frick, U., Hauser, S., Langguth, B., Rutschmann, R., Greenlee, M. W., Hajak, G., & Eichhammer, P. (2008) Neural correlates of symptom information in functional somatic syndromes: a fMRI study. *NeuroImage, 41*, 1336-1344.

P

Phelps, E. A. (2004) Human emotion and memory: interactions of the amygdala and hippocampal complex. *Current Opinion in Neurobiology 14*, 198–202.

S

Scaer, R. C. (2001). *The Body Bears The Burden*. The Hawthorn Medical Press.

Schwartz, J., and Begley, S. (2002). *The Mind and the Brain: Neuroplasticity and the Power of Mental Force*. Regan Books.

W

Wiest, G., Lehner-Baumgartner, E., & Baumgartner, C. (2006). Panic attacks in an individual with bilateral selective lesions of the amygdala. *Archives of Neurology, 63(12)*,1798-1801.

Williams, D.A., Gracely, R.H. (2006). Functional magnetic resonance imaging findings in fibromyalgia. *Arthritis Research and Therapy, 8(6)*, 224.